成人高等教育基础医学教材

大 学 英 语
Daxue Yingyu

（下册）

主　编　苏柳燕

上海科学技术出版社

图书在版编目(CIP)数据

大学英语.下册/苏柳燕主编.—上海:上海科学技术出
版社,2015.5(2016.5重印)
成人高等教育基础医学教材
ISBN 978－7－5478－2590－7

Ⅰ.①大... Ⅱ.①苏... Ⅲ.①英语－成人高等教育
－教材 Ⅳ.①H31

中国版本图书馆 CIP 数据核字(2015)第 059365 号

大学英语(下册)

主编 苏柳燕

上海世纪出版股份有限公司
上海 科 学 技 术 出 版 社 出版
(上海钦州南路 71 号 邮政编码 200235)
上海世纪出版股份有限公司发行中心发行
200001 上海福建中路 193 号 www.ewen.co
苏州望电印刷有限公司印刷
开本 787×1092 1/16 印张:8.25
字数:180 千字
2015 年 5 月第 1 版 2016 年 5 月第 3 次印刷
ISBN 978－7－5478－2590－7/H·18
定价:25.00 元

成人高等教育基础医学教材

编写委员会

■ **主任委员** 赵 群

■ **副主任委员** 陈金宝

■ **委 员** （以姓氏笔画为序）

于爱鸣	王 健	王丽宇	王怀良	王艳梅
王爱平	方 瑾	孔垂泽	田 静	邢 花
朱闻溪	刘 宇	刘俊亭	刘彩霞	汤艳清
孙田杰	孙海涛	苏兰若	苏柳燕	李 丹
李小寒	李红丽	李栢林	李福才	肖卫国
佟晓杰	邱 峰	邱雪杉	张 波	张东方
张喜轩	陈 迎	陈 磊	苑秀华	范 玲
罗恩杰	孟胜男	孟繁浩	赵 斌	赵成海
施万英	姜桂春	娄 岩	祝 峥	袁长季
钱 聪	徐东雨	徐甲芬	高丽红	曹 宇
蔡际群	翟效月	颜红炜	潘兴瑜	潘颖丽
薛辛东	魏敏杰			

■ **教材编写办公室**

刘 强 刘伟韬

成人高等教育基础医学教材

大学英语(下册)

编委会名单

■ **主　　编**　苏柳燕

■ **副 主 编**　王少鹏　陈　迎

■ **编　　者**　(以姓氏笔画为序)

　　　　　　王少鹏　王桂敏　苏柳燕　宋　阳

　　　　　　张　旭　陈　迎　赵丽娜

前　言

近年来，随着高等医学教育的迅速发展，全日制本科医药类教材建设得到了长足的进步，教材体系日益完善，品种迅速增多，质量逐渐提高。然而，针对成人护理学及药学专业高等教育教材，能够充分体现以教师为主导、以学生为主体、以学生自主学习为主模式的教材并不多。根据教育部《关于普通高等教育教材建设与改革的意见》的精神，为了进一步提高成人高等教育护理学及药学专业教材的质量，更好地把握 21 世纪成人高等教育护理学及药学内容和课程体系的改革方向，以中国医科大学为主，聘请了北京大学、复旦大学、中山大学、西安交通大学、江南大学、卫生部中日友好医院、辽宁中医药大学、沈阳药科大学、沈阳医学院和澳门理工学院等单位的专家编写了本系列教材，由上海科学技术出版社出版。本系列教材分为成人高等教育基础医学教材、成人高等教育护理学专业教材和成人高等教育药学专业教材，前者供护理学及药学专业学生使用，后两者分别为护理学及药学的专业教材。

本系列教材编排新颖、版式紧凑、层次清晰、结构合理。每章由三大部分组成：第一部分是导学，告知学生本章需要掌握的内容和重点难点，以方便教师教学和学生有目的地学习相关内容；第二部分是具体学习内容，力求体现科学性、适用性和易读性的特点；第三部分是复习题，便于学生课后复习，并附有答案。

本系列教材的使用对象主要为护理学及药学专业的高起本、高起专和专升本三个层次的学生。其中，对高起本和专升本层次的学习要求相同，对高起专层次的学习要求在每章导学部分予以说明。本系列教材中的基础医学教材也适用于其他相关医学专业。

除了教材外，我们还将通过中国医科大学网络教育平台（http://des.cmu.edu.cn）提供与教材配套的教学大纲、网络课件、电子教案、教学资源、网上练习、模拟测试等，为学生自主学习提供多种资源，建造一个立体化的学习环境。

为了确保本系列教材的编写进度和质量，我们成立了教材编写委员会。编写委员会主任委员由中国医科大学校长赵群教授担任，副主任委员由中国医科大学网络教育学院常务副院长陈金宝教授担任。编写委员会下设教材编写办公室，由刘强和刘伟韬同志负责各分册协调和部分编务工作等。教材部分绘图工作由齐亚力同志完成。

由于时间仓促，任务繁重，在教材编写中难免存在不足，恳请广大教师、学生和读者惠予指正，使本系列教材更臻完善，成为科学性强、教学效果更好、更符合现代成人高等教育要求的精品教材。

成人高等教育护理学及药学专业教材
编写委员会
2011 年 5 月

编 写 说 明

  《大学英语》(上、下册)教材顺应时代发展的需要,旨在遵循成人高等教育应用型人才的培养目标,针对从业人员继续教育的特点,本着学以致用的原则,紧紧围绕《大学英语》(B)考试大纲(2013年修订版)编写而成。在编写宗旨、单元设计、体裁及题材的选择上兼顾满足高升本、专升本学生的实际需要,全部内容适合高升本和专升本的学生使用。

  本书选材具有时代性、人文性和趣味性,同时还能激发学生的思考能力。在体裁上突出了实际应用性,涵盖了记叙文、议论文和说明文等。

  本书每单元由 Text A、Text B 和 Further Study 组成。每单元前均有 Guidance,告知学生本单元要掌握的重点及难点。Text A 和 Text B 属于正文学习,其后面的练习编写主要围绕课文理解,课文所涉及的句型、词汇及语法,旨在巩固提高所学的知识。Further Study 是延伸拓展学习,其中的 Communication Skills 总结归纳了日常生活中的交际用语;Grammar 是本书与同类书语法设计迥异的地方,本书打破了常规的语法讲解,取而代之的是对英语写作中易犯错误的语法的归纳讲解和练习。Writing 部分由浅及深,从句子翻译过渡到篇章写作,体现了语言学习循序渐进的输出功能。

  本教材实行主编负责制,书稿完成后由主编进行审定。从选材、编写到成稿,编者们耗费了大量时间和精力。但由于编者水平有限,本书在内容上难免疏漏和瑕疵,敬请读者海涵,不吝赐教。

《大学英语》编委会

2014 年 8 月

Content

Unit One
Friendship

Guidance

1. This unit consists of Text A, Text B and Further Study. **Text A** reveals what real friendship is by telling a true story about two friends who have sustained the test of time and distance without faltering. **Text B** gives us advice on how to heal a broken friendship. **Further Study** focuses on communication skills in terms of expressing thanks and the possible responses.

2. By learning this unit, students will be able to master the structure of the texts, new words, phrases and expressions. Students will improve their understanding of grammatical structures, reading comprehension and enlarge their vocabulary by doing the relevant exercises. Meanwhile, they will gain better understanding on *Friendship*.

3. **Further Study** aims to improve students' skills for communication. By doing the exercises, students will know the differences in communication between Chinese and Westerners. They will perform well in everyday conversation and writing by doing this part.

- Real Friends
- How to Heal a Friendship

> No matter how strong you are, how notable your attainments, you have enduring significance only in your relationship to others.
>
> — Ziegler Edward

■■ Text A   Real Friends

Anonymous

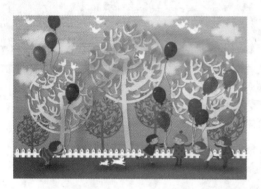

I grew up in Jamaica Plain, an urban community located on the outskirts of Boston, Massachusetts. In the 1940's it was a wholesome, quaint little community. It was my home and I loved it; back then I thought I would never leave. My best friend Rose and I used to collectively dream[1] about raising a family of our own someday. We had it all planned out to live next door to one another.

Our dream remained alive through grade school[2], high school, and even beyond. Rose was my maid of honor[3] when I got married in 1953 to the love of my life, Dick. Meanwhile, Dick aspired to be an officer in the Marines and I fully supported his ambitions. I realized that he might be stationed far away from Jamaica Plain, but I told him I would relocate and adjust.

So, in 1955 Dick was stationed in Alaska and we relocated. Rose was sad to see me leave, but wished me the best of luck[4]. Rose and I remained in touch for a few years via periodic phone calls but after a while we lost track of one another. Back in the 1950's it was a lot more difficult to stay in touch with someone over a long distance, especially if you were relocating every few years.

I thought of her several times over the years. Once in the mid 1960's when I was visiting the Greater Boston area[5], I tried to determine her whereabout, but my search turned up empty-handed. Jamaica Plain had changed drastically in the 10 years I was gone. My family had moved out of the area, as did many of the people I used to know. Rose was nowhere to be found.

Fifty-two years passed and we never spoke. I've raised a family of five, all of whom now have families of their own, and Dick passed away a few years ago. Basically, a lifetime has passed. Now here I am at the doorstep to my 80th birthday and I receive a random phone call on an idle Wednesday afternoon. "Hello?" I said. "Hi, Natalie. It's Rose," the voice on the other end replied. "It's been so long. I don't know if you remember me, but we used to be best friends in Jamaica Plain when we were kids," she said.

We haven't seen each other yet, but we have spent countless hours on the phone catching up on 52 years of our lives. The interesting thing is that even after 52 years of separation our personalities and interests are still extremely similar. We both share a passion for several hobbies that we picked up independently after we lost touch with one another, which is really strange considering the circumstances.

Her husband passed away a few years ago as well, but she mailed me several photographs of her family that were taken over the years. It's so crazy, just looking at the photos and listening to her describe her family reminds me of my own. It feels like we led fairly similar lives.

I don't think the numerous similarities between our two lives are a coincidence. Real friends have two things in common: a compatible personality and a strong-willed character. The compatible personality is what initiates the connection between two people and a strong-willed character at both ends is what maintains the connection. If those two ingredients are present in a friendship, the friendship is for real, and can thus sustain the tests of time and prolonged absence without faltering.

New Words

community /kəˈmjuːnɪtɪ/	*n.* a group of people living together or united by shared interests, religion, nationality, etc. 社区;团体
located /ləʊˈkeɪtɪd/	*adj.* situated in a particular spot or position 位于,处于
outskirts /ˈaʊtskɜːts/	*n.* the parts of a city or town that are farthest away from its centre 市郊,郊区
wholesome /ˈhəʊls(ə)m/	*adj.* ① conducive to or characteristic of physical or moral well-being 有益健康的 ② sound or exhibiting soundness in body or mind 健全的
quaint /kweɪnt/	*adj.* attractive because it is old-fashioned 古雅的
collectively /kəˈlektɪvlɪ/	*adv.* in conjunction with or combined 共同地,集体地
aspire /əˈspaɪə/	*vi.* to have a strong desire to achieve something 渴望,向往,有志于
Marines /məˈriːns/	*n.* members of a body of troops trained to serve on land or at sea 海军陆战队
station /ˈsteɪʃn/	*vt.* to be send to a place to do a job or to work for a period of time 派驻,驻扎
	n. (the building or buildings at) a place where the stated public vehicles regularly stop so that passengers can get on and off, goods can be loaded, etc. 车站
relocate /riːlə(ʊ)ˈkeɪt/	*vt. & vi.* to move or establish in a new location (使)迁移;(使)重新安置
via /ˈvaɪə/	*prep.* ① by means of or using 通过,凭借 ② traveling or sent through (a place) on the way 经由
periodic /ˌpɪərɪˈɒdɪk/	*adj.* happening fairly regularly 周期的,定期的
distance /ˈdɪst(ə)ns/	*n.* amount of space between two points or places 距离,间距
whereabout /ˈwerəbaʊt/	*n.* the place where a particular person or thing may be found 行踪,下落
	adv. about where or near what place 在何处,在哪里
empty-handed /ˌemptiːˈhændɪd/	*adj.* ① having acquired or gained nothing 一无所获的 ② carrying nothing in the hands 空手的,徒手的

drastically /'dræstɪkəlɪ/   *adv*. in a drastic manner 大幅度地;彻底地;激烈地

basically /'beɪsɪk(ə)lɪ/   *adv*. with regard to what is most important and basic, or in reality 基本上,根本上,本质上

lifetime /'laɪftaɪm/   *n*. the length of time that someone is alive 一生,终生

doorstep /'dɔːstep/   *n*. a step in front of a door on the outside of a building 门阶

random /'rændəm/   *adj*. ① happening at any time or unplanned 任意的,无计划的 ② (in statistics) having an equal chance of success (统计学)随机的

idle /'aɪd(ə)l/   *adj*. ① not working or operating productively 空闲的,闲着的 ② lazy, wasting time 懒散的,无所事事的

separation /sepə'reɪʃ(ə)n/   *n*. the act of dividing or disconnecting 分离,分开

personality /pɜːsə'nælɪtɪ/   *n*. characteristics and qualities of a person seen as a whole 个性,人格

passion /'pæʃ(ə)n/   *n*. ① a strong liking or enthusiasm for sth 爱好,酷爱 ② strong, deep, often uncontrollable feeling 激情,热情

independently /ɪndɪ'pend(ə)ntlɪ/   *adv*. on your own, or without outside help, or apart from others 独立地;自立地;各自地

circumstance /'sɜːkəmst(ə)ns/   *n*. the conditions which affect what happens 情况,情形,形势

mail /meɪl/   *vt*. to send a letter or package to someone by putting it in a postbox or taking it to a post office 邮寄
   n. ① the public service or system by which letters and parcels are collected and delivered 邮政,邮政系统 ② letters and parcels that are delivered 邮件,信件,邮包

numerous /'njuːm(ə)rəs/   *adj*. existing or present in large numbers 许多的

similarity /sɪmə'lærətɪ/   *n*. features that things have which make them similar to each other 相似点,类似的地方

coincidence /kəʊ'ɪnsɪd(ə)ns/   *n*. occurrence of similar events or circumstances at the same time by chance 巧合

compatible /kəm'pætɪb(ə)l/   *adj*. able to exist together, live together, or be used together 可并存的,兼容的

strong-willed /'strɒŋ'wɪld/   *adj*. having a determined will 意志坚强的,固执己见的

initiate /ɪ'nɪʃɪeɪt/   *vt*. to start or cause something to happen 使开始,发起

maintain /meɪn'teɪn/   *vt*. to continue to have something and do not let it stop or grow weaker 维持,保持

ingredient /ɪn'griːdɪənt/   *n*. ① one of the essential parts of a situation 要素,因素 ② any of the things that are formed into a mixture when making something, especially in cooking 成分,(烹调的)原料

sustain /sə'steɪn/   *vt*. ① to continue or maintain something for a period of time 保持 ② to support someone by giving help, strength, or encouragement 支撑

test /test/   *n*. ① an event or situation that reveals the qualities or effectiveness of a person or thing 考验 ② a number of questions, exercises, etc., for measuring one's skill, cleverness or knowledge of a particular subject 测验　③ a deliberate action or experiment to find out how well something works 试验

prolonged /prə'lɒŋd/　　　*adj*. continuing for a long time, or for longer than expected 持续很久的,延长的

falter /'fɔːltə/　　　*vi*. ① to lose power or strength in an uneven way, or no longer makes much progress 衰退,变弱　② to hesitate or pause when speaking, because you are unsure about what you are saying or are upset (说话)迟疑,吞吞吐吐,支吾

Phrases and Expressions

one another	互相;彼此
after a while	不久以后
lose track of	失去联系
turn up	出现;(被)发现;(被)证明是
catch up on	赶上;弥补
pick up	拾起;学会;获得;(开车)接
pass away	去世;停止
remind ... of	使……想起
have ... in common	与……有共同之处
for real	真正的;确实的

Text Notes

1. used to do 意为"过去经常做……",其中 to 是不定式符号,而不是介词,所以其后只接动词原形,不能接名词。例如:He used to live in Paris. 他过去一直住在巴黎。而 be used to doing 意为"习惯于……",其中 to 是介词,所以其后要接名词或动名词,不能接动词原形。例如:He is used to looking after himself. 他已习惯于自己照顾自己。另外,be used to do 是动词 use 的被动语态结构,意为"被用来做……",其中 to 为不定式符号,其后要接动词原形。例如:A hammer is used to drive in nails. 锤子是用来钉钉子的。

2. grade school 在美式英语中意为"小学",与 elementary school, grammar school, primary school 含义相同。例如:He went to grade school in New York and high school in Chicago. 他是在纽约上的小学,芝加哥上的中学。

3. maid of honor 意为"伴娘""首席女傧相",西方人对于伴郎与伴娘通常会慎重选择,伴娘往往从新娘的未婚好友或姐妹中选出,通常只能有一位,另外新娘在婚礼上还可能有三至四位 bridesmaid (女傧相)作陪(但地位都不及伴娘崇高),当新娘邀请自己的某位好友或姐妹做伴娘时,对于被邀请人来说,意味着信任与深厚的感情,也确实是一种荣耀。另外,best man 为"伴郎"。

4. wish sb. the best of luck 表示"祝……好运""祝……一切顺利"。例如:I wish you the best of luck in all your endeavors. 我希望好运永远伴随你的左右。

5. the Greater Boston (area)意为"大波士顿""大波士顿地区"。波士顿是美国历史的摇篮,自 1620 年"五月花号"帆船从英国载来第一代移民,波士顿就在美国历史上扮演重要的角色,它是美国最早建立的城市之一,也是美国新英格兰地区最大的城市(美国东北六州统称新英格兰地区)。波

士顿是新英格兰地区政治和文化中心，目前有 50 多所大学和学院，包括著名的哈佛大学和麻省理工学院。波士顿和周围众多卫星城镇组成的大都会统称大波士顿地区。

Text Comprehension

Please choose the best answers to the following questions according to the text.

1. The reason why Dick and I left Jamaica Plain is that _____ .

    A. my friendship with Rose was broken

    B. Dick was stationed by the Marines in Alaska and we relocated

    C. we were fed up with life in Jamaica Plain

    D. the Jamaica Plain changed drastically

2. What does the word "periodic" mean in Para. 3?

    A. Regular.   B. Chronic.   C. Rare.   D. Timely.

3. Rose and I remained in touch for a few years but later we lost track of one another, because _____ .

    A. I forgot Rose's telephone number

    B. I did not give Rose my home address

    C. both of us were so occupied with work that we could hardly spare any time for social activities

    D. it was difficult to keep in touch with people over a long distance at that time, and even worse, Dick and I often relocated

4. After 52 years of separation, Rose and I _____ .

    A. can hardly find anything in common

    B. forget all about each other

    C. still have similar personalities and interests

    D. fail to choose any topic to talk about

5. According to the author, real friendship _____ .

    A. ends for many different reasons

    B. withstands the test of time and distance

    C. is based on mutual understanding and trust

    D. is often more intense in an individual's childhood than in his adulthood

Vocabulary and Structure

Please choose the best answer for each of the following sentences.

1. _____ education is the instruction that occurs when the instructor and students are separated by distance or time, or both.

    A. Separation   B. Distance

    C. Length   D. Gap

2. The winners will be selected at _____ from the correct answers received.

    A. formal   B. casual

    C. idle   D. random

3. Under no _____ should we be reckless of consequence and make hasty decisions.

A. instance   B. circumstance
C. situation   D. environment

4. Despite _____ attempts to diet, her weight soared.

A. numerous   B. numerable
C. much   D. continuous

5. The new system will be _____ with existing equipment.

A. capable   B. controllable
C. compatible   D. considerable

Comprehensive Exercise

There are five incomplete sentences in the following passage. Read the passage and choose the word that best fits into the passage. Do remember each word can be used only once.

> A. to   B. same   C. of   D. as   E. on

Just __1__ a band or gang of superheroes needs members who have different talents and powers, a circle of friends should have exactly the same thing. It's important to have diversity and to be able __2__ look for support from a variety __3__ sources. They also help us to keep broader perspective __4__ life.

You need different types of friends in the __5__ way that you need food from different food groups. Different types of friends serve different purposes and nourish and enrich our lives in different ways.

Translation

Please translate the following sentences into Chinese.

1. The United Nations has appealed for help from the international community.
2. He has spent a lifetime fighting against racism and prejudice.
3. Separation from his friends made him very sad.
4. His passion for reading never deserted him.
5. The house costs a fortune to maintain.

■■ Text B   How to Heal a Friendship

Anonymous

Jessica and Joyce were best friends in ninth grade. They did almost everything together. Then one day, after a misunderstanding, Joyce stopped talking to Jessica. For more than three months, Joyce refused to talk to Jessica or answer her notes. "During that time, I found out what an important friend she was," Jessica says. "I couldn't even concentrate when I was studying. I just thought about how to mend our friendship." The next semester, Jessica tried again. This time, Joyce was willing to work it out. It took some

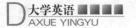
time and effort, but the friendship was healed.

Most of us have suffered the pain of broken friendships. But the good news is that[1] most friendships can be mended.

Oxford professor Michael Argyle recently finished a 15-year study that explored what makes people happy. He found that the key to happiness is having one close relationship and a network of friends. Other studies show that our social connections make us healthier and more resilient to stress. Maintaining long-lasting, healthy friendships is worth[2] the effort!

If there's a broken friendship you'd like to mend, try the following advice.

Give your friend the benefit of the doubt.[3]

It's easy to assume the worst[4]. But if a friend has hurt you, he may not even realize he's done so.

Matt, an American doctoral student, remembers two friendships broken by hurtful words. Both relationships were later healed. "It's probably true that if someone hurts you, they should have known better[5]", Matt says. "But the fact is we are all human and we mess things up. You need to give people the benefit of the doubt because you will need that, as well."

Take the initiative to communicate with your friend.

If you've been hurt, your instinct is probably to pull away and protect yourself. But if you do this, the friendship will likely die.

"You need to reach out," says 20-year-old Jamie, who has restored several broken friendships. "Friendships get broken when trust is lost. Both friends need to reach out and demonstrate they are trustworthy."

Be the first to apologize. Even if you were hurt, apologize for anything you did wrong. Give up your right to be proven right. Otherwise the conflict won't be forgotten, as it should be.

Walk through the conflict together.

Start by trying to see things from your friend's point of view. Talk about the problems openly but kindly.

At first, Jessica didn't understand why Joyce stopped talking to her. Then Joyce finally explained that Jessica's teasing bothered her. "I finally found out she was angry because I teased her in front of the boys in our class," Jessica explained. Jessica meant nothing by her teasing and thought it shouldn't bother Joyce. But when she accepted that it was embarrassing to Joyce, she stopped. Then their friendship could heal.

Nicole and Michelle had been best friends since preschool. But in college, Michelle suddenly pulled away. "We didn't talk to each other for a while, then tried to reconcile," Nicole says, "but we're just polite acquaintances now."

It's normal for friendships to change. Often two friends just drift apart. Problems come when one friend tries to hang on while the other friend lets go. If your friend isn't willing to work things out, accept it and move on. But if you are able to reconcile, you'll have a friendship that's tried-and-true!

New Words

heal /hiːl/ — *vt. & vi.* ① to become healthy and normal again 治愈,痊愈 ② to put something such as a rift or a wound right so that people are friendly or happy again （使）（裂痕、创伤）弥合,（使）和好

misunderstanding /ˌmɪsʌndəˈstændɪŋ/ — *n.* a failure to understand something properly, for example a situation or a person's remarks 误解,误会

refuse /rɪˈfjuːz/ — *vt. & vi.* to state one's strong unwillingness to accept or do something 拒绝

note /nəʊt/ — *n.* ① a short letter 便条 ② short written record to aid the memory 记录,笔记

concentrate /ˈkɒns(ə)ntreɪt/ — *vt. & vi.* ① to focus all one's attention on something 集中（心思）,专心 ② come or bring together in a small area 集中

mend /mend/ — *vt. & vi.* ① to repair something that is broken or not working, so that it works properly or can be used 修理,修补 ② to heal or recover （使）康复;（使）痊愈

semester /sɪˈmestə/ — *n.* one of the two main periods into which the year is divided in colleges and universities in some countries 学期

willing /ˈwɪlɪŋ/ — *adj.* fairly happy or enthusiastic about doing something 乐意的,心甘情愿的

effort /ˈefət/ — *n.* the use of physical strength or power of the mind, or the earnest and conscientious activity intended to do or accomplish something 努力

explore /ɪkˈsplɔː/ — *vt.* ① to think about or comment on something in detail, in order to assess it carefully 探讨,研究 ② to travel around a place to find out what it is like 探测,勘察,考察

relationship /rɪˈleɪʃ(ə)nʃɪp/ — *n.* the way in which two things are connected 联系,关系

network /ˈnetwɜːk/ — *n.* a large number of people or institutions that have a connection with each other or work together as a system 网络

social /ˈsəʊʃ(ə)l/ — *adj.* ① relating to society or to the way society is organized 社会的 ② relating to leisure activities that involve meeting other people 社交的

connection /kəˈnekʃn/ — *n.* a relationship between two things, people, or groups 联系,关系

resilient /rɪˈzɪlɪənt/ — *adj.* strong and not easily damaged by being hit, stretched, or squeezed 有弹性的

stress /stres/ — *n.* pressure caused by the problems of living, too much work, etc. 压力

long-lasting /ˈlɔːŋlɑːstɪŋ/ — *adj.* lasting for a long time 持久的

assume /əˈsjuːm/ — *vt.* ① to take to be the case or to be true or accept without verification or proof 假定，认为　② to take on titles, offices, duties, responsibilities 承担，担任，就职

doctoral /ˈdɒkt(ə)r(ə)l/　*adj*. of or relating to a doctor or doctorate 博士的，博士学位的

hurtful /ˈhɜːtfl/　*adj*. causing hurt or harmful to living things 伤感情的，有害的

communicate /kəˈmjuːnɪkeɪt/　*vi*. to share or exchange information with someone, for example by speaking, writing, or using equipment 交流，沟通

instinct /ˈɪnstɪŋ(k)t/　*n*. ① the natural tendency that a person or animal has to behave or react in a particular way 本能　② a feeling, rather than an opinion or idea based on facts, that something is the case 直觉

protect /prəˈtekt/　*vt*. to prevent someone or something from being harmed or damaged 保护

likely /ˈlaɪklɪ/　*adj*. indicating that something is probably the case or will probably happen in a particular situation 可能的

　　adv. with considerable certainty or without much doubt 很可能

restore /rɪˈstɔː/　*vt. & vi*. to cause someone or something to exist again or to be in the previous condition or place once again （使）恢复，（使）修复，（使）复原

demonstrate /ˈdemənstreɪt/　*vt*. ① to make a fact clear to people 证明　② to show people how something works or how to do something 展示

　　vi. to march or gather somewhere to show one's opposition to or support for something 游行示威

trustworthy /ˈtrʌs(t)wɜːðɪ/　*adj*. reliable, responsible, and can be trusted completely 可信赖的，可靠的

apologize /əˈpɒlədʒaɪz/　*vi*. to acknowledge faults or shortcomings or failing 道歉，认错

prove /pruːv/　*vt. & vi*. to show by means of argument or evidence that something is definitely true 证明（是）

otherwise /ˈʌðəwaɪz/　*adv*. in another or different way, or in other or different respects 否则，另外，在其他方面

　　conj. if conditions were different, or if not 否则，要不然

conflict /ˈkɒnflɪkt/　*n*. ① serious disagreement and argument about something important between two people or groups 争执，分歧　② fighting between countries or groups of people （军事）冲突，战斗

openly /ˈəʊpənlɪ/　*adv*. without hiding any facts or one's feelings 公开地

bother /ˈbɒðə/　*vt. & vi*. to cause annoyance, or disturb, especially by minor irritations （使）烦恼，（使）不安

tease /tiːz/　*vt*. to laugh at or make jokes about someone in order to embarrass, annoy, or upset them 嘲笑，取笑

embarrassing /ɪmˈbærəsɪŋ/　*adj*. making someone feel shy or ashamed 令人尴尬的

preschool /ˈpriːskuːl/　*n*. a school for children between the ages of 2 and 5 or 6 （两岁至五六岁孩子的）学前班，学前学校

　　adj. relating to the care and education of children before they reach the age when they have to go to school 入学前的，学龄

前的

reconcile /'rek(ə)nsaɪl/	*vt*. to make them become friends again after a quarrel or disagreement 使……和解
acquaintance /ə'kweɪnt(ə)ns/	*n*. ① someone who you have met and know slightly，but not well 相识之人　② a relationship less intimate than friendship 认识，相识　③ personal knowledge or information about someone or something 了解，熟悉
normal /'nɔːm(ə)l/	*adj*. usual and ordinary，and in accordance with what people expect 正常的，通常的，平常的
tried-and-true /'traɪdən'truː/	*adj*. tested and proved to be reliable 经过检验而可靠的，靠得住的

Phrases and Expressions

work . . . out	解决……；算出……
mess . . . up	把……搞糟；把……弄乱
take the initiative	采取主动
pull away	离开；疏远；脱身
reach out	伸出(手)
give up	放弃；让出
drift apart	(逐渐)疏远；漂离；各奔东西
hang on	坚持；抓紧；不挂断
let go	放手；松手；放开；释放
move on	继续前进；往前走

Text Notes

1. good news 表示"好消息""喜讯"，the good news is that . . .可以翻译为"好消息是……""令人欣慰的是……""值得高兴的是……"。例如：The good news is that expert help is now available. 令人欣慰的是现在可以获得专家的帮助。

2. worth 作形容词时，只能在句子中作表语，表示"值(多少钱)""相当于……的价值""值得做……"(主动结构表示被动意义)，其后接名词或动名词的主动形式。例如：A local jeweler says the pearl is worth at least＄500. 一位本地珠宝商说这颗珍珠至少值500美元。Although at times，learning a language was frustrating，it was well worth the effort. 尽管学习一门外语时常遭遇挫折，但付出的努力还是很值得的。The novel is worth reading. 这部小说值得一读。

3. the benefit of the doubt 表示"无罪推定""假定某人无罪"，指在没有证据之前，先假定某人无罪或相信某人的清白。例如：A suspected criminal must have the benefit of the doubt until we're certain he's guilty. 在未能确定一名嫌疑犯有罪之前，他应该被视为是无罪的。在此文中，本句可译为"在未经证实之前，愿意假定你的朋友是无辜的"。

4. assume the worst 在文中表示"假设最坏的情况""作最坏的假设""往最坏处想"。例如：Rational policymakers must assume the worst. 理性的政策制定者必须作最坏的打算。

5. should have done 为虚拟语气，表示与过去事实相反的虚拟假设，意为"本应该做(而没做)……"。文中此处 they should have known better，译为"他们本应该更清楚""他们本应该更明白"，即"他们本应该知道伤人的言语会破坏友谊(而不说伤害朋友的话)"。

Text Comprehension

Please read the following statements and mark T/F according to the text.

1. Jessica's friendship with Joyce could never be healed because of a misunderstanding.
   A. T   B. F

2. Happiness has nothing to do with one's relationship with friends.
   A. T   B. F

3. If it's not your fault，you don't need to apologize or prove yourself right to your friend.
   A. T   B. F

4. Trying to see things from your friend's point of view is conducive to healing a friendship.
   A. T   B. F

5. Best friends could be polite acquaintances if they are not willing to work things out and reconcile.
   A. T   B. F

Vocabulary and Structure

Please choose the best answer for each of the following sentences.

1. The quarrel originated in a _____ . （understand）
2. He was _____ to make any sacrifice for peace. （will）
3. Scientists have established a _____ between cholesterol levels and heart disease. （connect）
4. Someone allergic to milk is _____ to react to cheese. （like）
5. A friend might be an _____ or an intimate companion that one has known since childhood. （acquaint）

Translation

Please translate the following passage into Chinese.

Studies show that the key to happiness is having one close relationship and a network of friends. Our social connections make us healthier and more resilient to stress. Maintaining long-lasting，healthy friendships is worth the effort!

⠿ Further Study

（Thanks and Responses）

Communication Skills

感谢与应答（Thanks and Responses）：包括接受对方的帮助、邀请、款待或礼物、拜访或电话问候等多种情况，在家人、朋友、上下级、甚至陌生人之间的使用都极为广泛。

Key Sentences

◆ Expressing thanks
○ Thank you (very much).
○ Thanks (a lot).
○ Thank you for your help.
○ It's very kind (thoughtful) of you.
○ How kind (thoughtful) of you!
○ (I'm very) Much obliged (to you).
○ I'm really very grateful to you.
○ I shall always feel indebted to you.
○ Thank you all the same.
◆ Possible responses
○ My pleasure.
○ Not at all.
○ You're welcome.
○ No trouble at all. I'm always glad to help you.
○ I'm so glad you like it.
○ Sure thing.
○ It's been a pleasure.
○ I'm very glad to have been of help to you.
○ I'm afraid I haven't done as much as I should.

Practice

1. — Thanks for your help.

  — _____

  A. My pleasure.   B. Quite right.   C. Never mind.   D. Don't thank me.

2. — Thank you so much for your lovely gift.

  — _____

  A. Never mind.   B. Please don't say so.
  C. I'm glad you like it.   D. No, it's not so good.

3. — Thank you for your invitation.

  — _____

  A. It doesn't matter.   B. It's a pleasure.
  C. I'll appreciate it.   D. It's a small thing.

4. — Thank you for calling.

  — _____

  A. Don't mention it.   B. Nice talking to you.
  C. That's fine.   D. Call back again.

5. — It's been a wonderful evening. Thank you very much.

  — _____

A．Just so-so.　　　B．No，thanks.　　　C．My pleasure.　　　D．It's OK.

Grammar

动词时态(Tense of Verb)：

　　英语中不同时间和方式发生的动作或状态要用谓语动词的不同形式来表示，这种表示动作或状态发生时间和方式的动词形式称作动词时态。

　　时态是动词的"时"和"体"的组合。"时"分为现在、过去、将来和过去将来；而"体"分为一般、进行、完成和完成进行。

　　其中，进行体用来表示现在、过去或将来的某一时间正在进行的动作；而完成体通常用来表示现在、过去或将来的某一时间已经完成的动作。

	一般	进行	完成	完成进行
现在	一般现在时 do / does	现在进行时 am / is / are doing	现在完成时 have / has done	现在完成进行时 have / has been doing
过去	一般过去时 did	过去进行时 was / were doing	过去完成时 had done	过去完成进行时 had been doing
将来	一般将来时 will do	将来进行时 will be doing	将来完成时 will have done	将来完成进行时 will have been doing
过去将来	过去将来时 would do	过去将来进行时 would be doing	过去将来完成时 would have done	过去将来完成进行时 would have been doing

Practice

1. I first met Simon three years ago. She _____ at a university at that time.
   A．has worked
   B．was working
   C．has been working
   D．had worked

2. — Is this raincoat yours?
   — No，mine _____ there behind the door.
   A．is hanging　　　B．hangs　　　C．has hung　　　D．hung

3. My watch _____ at nine o'clock, but now it _____ .
   A．went；stopped
   B．went；is stopping
   C．was going；stopped
   D．was going；has stopped

4. By the time you arrive in London，we _____ in Europe for two weeks.
   A．shall stay
   B．will have stayed
   C．have stayed
   D．have been staying

5. Mrs. White became a teacher in 1985. She _____ for twenty years by next summer.
   A．will teach
   B．has been teaching
   C．would have taught
   D．will have been teaching

Writing

邀请信(Letter of Invitation):邀请信是邀请亲朋好友或知名人士、专家等参加聚会、婚礼、会议、宴请等活动时所发出的请约性书信。在国际交往以及日常的各种社交活动中,这类书信使用广泛。英文邀请信可分为两种:一种是正规的邀请信,又称请柬(invitation card),其格式严谨而固定,一般适用于较庄重严肃的场合;另一种是一般邀请信,适用于非正式场合的邀请,通常邀请人同被邀请人之间关系较为熟悉,因而这种邀请信具有语言简短、热情等特点。

一、邀请信的主要内容

包括:邀请对象、活动时间、活动地点、活动内容、询问是否接受邀请等。在邀请信中应具体写明:

1. 活动名称及目的:写明邀请对方参加什么活动,以及邀请的原因及目的等。

2. 活动细节及注意事项:写明活动安排的细节及需要告诉对方的注意事项。诸如时间、地点、参加人员、人数,需要做哪些准备及服饰要求等。

3. 回函要求:希望被邀请人收信后对是否接受邀请给予答复,要在请柬上注明 R.S.V.P 或 r.s.v.p.字样,意为"请答复"。有时为方便联系,可留下邀请人或联系人的电话号码或其他联系方式。

二、邀请信常用句型:

(一)正规邀请信 / 请柬

1. May I have the honor of your company at dinner? 敬备菲酌,恭请光临。

2. Request the pleasure of ... 恭请……

3. We have decided to have a party in honor of the occasion. 为此我们决定举办一场晚会。

4. The reception will be held in ... on... 招待会定于……在……举行。

5. I hope you are not too busy to come. 我期望您在百忙中光临。

6. We sincerely hope you can attend. 我们期待您的光临。

7. Please confirm your participation at your earliest convenience. 是否参加,请早日告之。

8. The favor of a reply is requested. 敬赐复函。

(二)一般邀请信

1. I am writing to invite you to ... 我写信是想邀请你……

2. I think it would be a great idea if you could participate in ... 我想如果你能参加……将是一个非常好的主意。

3. We would be looking forward to your coming with great pleasure. 我们很高兴地期待着你的到来。

4. Would you please drop me a line to let me know if you can come to ...? 你可以写封短信来告诉我你能否来……吗?

5. I would like to meet you there and please let me know your decision soon. 我希望能在那见到你,请早点让我知道你的决定。

Practice

Instructions:Prof. Robin 是研究英国文学的知名学者,你作为英语学院的院长助理,请你代表院长写一封正式的邀请信,邀请 Prof. Robin 来你所在学院进行短期访问并为师生作一次讲座。

Unit Two
Sports

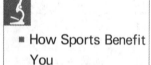

- How Sports Benefit You
- Father's Eyes

Guidance

1. This unit consists of Text A, Text B and Further Study. **Text A** tells us in which way sports benefit us. **Text B** introduces a story about a skinny boy who loved football with all his heart and succeeded after suffering and practising a lot. **Further Study** focuses on communication skills.

2. By learning this unit, students will be able to master the structure of the texts, new words, phrases and expressions. Students will improve their understanding of grammatical structures, reading comprehension and broaden their vocabulary by doing the relevant exercises. Meanwhile, they will gain better understanding of *Sports* and *Sports Spirit*.

3. **Further Study** aims to improve students' skills for communication. By doing the exercises, students will know how to make apologies. They will perform well in everyday conversation and writing by doing this part.

> Sports serve society by providing vivid examples of excellence.
>
> — George F. Will

▪▪ Text A   How Sports Benefit You

Anonymous

Playing sports is something most of us love, isn't it? Undoubtedly, sports are a fun activity but they offer several health benefits too. Playing some sport regularly goes a long way in maintaining your physical and mental well-being.[1] Sports help enhance your personality.

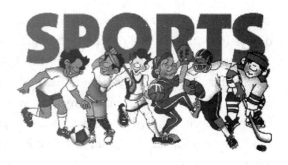

They are a good source of both exercise and entertainment.

Sports serve as an excellent physical exercise. Those who play sports have a more positive body image than those who do not. Sports often involve physical activities like running, jumping, stretching and moving about, which turn out to be a good body workout. Playing sports is energy put to good use[2]. Engaging in sports since an early age strengthens your bones and muscles and tones your body. It helps you increase your stamina and endurance. Sports that involve jumping and stretching help increase height, for example basketball. Games that involve running, kicking or throwing a ball help strengthen the arms and legs, for example soccer and cricket. Swimming provides a full body workout. Thus sports provide the body with complete exercise and engaging in sports directly translates into overall fitness.

Research shows that sports improve Math skills in children. Sports that involve aiming and hitting skills, for example, tennis, badminton, baseball and cricket help them increase focus. They help develop leadership qualities and foster team spirit in kids. They involve competition; they involve winning and losing. This exposes children to both aspects of life, successes and failures. Sports build a competitive spirit in children and teach them to be participative irrespective of[3] whether the result is victory or defeat. Playing sports teaches them to accept both successes and failures with a positive spirit.

Playing sports is very beneficial for the development of social skills. Sports teach you to interact with people, communicate with them and collaborate as a team. Sports foster collective thinking and harness your planning and delegation skills too. Sports build confidence. Winning a game gives you a sense of accomplishment, which boosts your confidence further.

Sports make you happy. I know anyone would agree with this. Jumping about, running around, racing to get ahead, hitting, throwing, bouncing, kicking (the ball, I mean!), shouting, clapping, cheering, falling and standing up again... all a part of playing sports. And there is no match to the happiness this brings. They give you the high by increasing the production of endorphins in the brain. In other words, sports are a form of exercise which generates happiness molecules in your body[4], thus restoring your mental health. Playing sports, you can't be sad. In fact, they bust the sorrow and the stress. Sports generate a positive energy in you, around you.

Playing sports reduces several health risks. As sports serve as an excellent form of exercise, it won't come as a surprise that they offer health benefits like lowering blood pressure, maintaining blood sugar and cholesterol levels and reducing other health risks.[5] Yes, if you are playing a sport regularly, you are at a lesser risk of developing diabetes or heart diseases. Playing sports reduces the risk of hypertension and several other stress-related disorders. Research shows that people who play sports regularly can deal with stresses and strains in a better way. Those who engage in sports activities are less prone to depression, anxiety and other psychological disorders.

Regular exercise that is achieved through sports leads to an improvement in the overall health thus improving quality of life. Sports are a good combination of recreation and exercise. They improve your physical and psychological health; physical because sports involve exercise and psychological because playing is something you enjoy, it's something that relaxes your mind. Something so advantageous is worth investing time in. So go hit the ground today.

New Words

undoubtedly /ʌnˈdaʊtɪdlɪ/	*adv*. with certainty 确实地;无庸置疑地
maintain /meɪnˈteɪn/	*vt*. ① to keep in a certain state, position, or activity 维持 ② to state categorically 主张
well-being /ˌwelˈbiːɪŋ/	*n*. a contented state of being happy and healthy and prosperous 幸福;康乐
enhance /ɪnˈhɑːns/	*vt*. to increase or make better 提高;加强;增加
personality /ˌpɜːsəˈnælɪtɪ/	*n*. the complex of all the attributes that characterize a unique individual 个性;品格
entertainment /ˌentəˈteɪnm(ə)nt/	*n*. an activity that is diverting and that holds the attention 娱乐;消遣;款待
stretch /stretʃ/	*v*. ① to occupy a large, elongated area 延伸 ② to extend one's limbs or muscles, or the entire body 伸展;张开
workout /ˈwɜːkaʊt/	*n*. the activity of exerting your muscles in various ways to keep fit 锻炼
strengthen /ˈstreŋθ(ə)n/	*v*. to make strong or stronger 加强;巩固
stamina /ˈstæmɪnə/	*n*. enduring strength and energy 毅力;精力;活力;持久力
endurance /ɪnˈdjʊər(ə)ns/	*n*. the power to withstand hardship or stress 忍耐力;忍耐;持久;耐久
cricket /ˈkrɪkɪt/	*n*. ① a game played with a ball and bat by two teams of 11 players 板球;板球运动 ② leaping insect 蟋蟀
provide /prəˈvaɪd/	*v*. to furnish with 提供;装备
overall /ˈəʊvərɔːl/	*adj*. & *adv*. including everything 全部的;全体的;总的说来
fitness /ˈfɪtnəs/	*n*. ① good physical condition 健康 ② the condition of being suitable 适当;适合性
badminton /ˈbædmɪnt(ə)n/	*n*. a game played on a court with light long-handled rackets used to volley a shuttlecock over a net 羽毛球
leadership /ˈliːdəʃɪp/	*n*. the activity of leading 领导能力
foster /ˈfɒstə/	*v*. ① to help develop 培养 ② to help grow 养育,抚育
	adj. providing or receiving nurture or parental care though not related by blood or legal ties 收养的;养育的
competition /ˌkɒmpɪˈtɪʃ(ə)n/	*n*. the act of competing as for profit or a prize 竞争;比赛;竞赛

aspect /ˈæspekt/ — *n*. a distinct feature or element in a problem 方面;方向

participative /pɑːˈtɪsɪpeɪtɪv/ — *adj*. being participating 参与的;分担的

irrespective /ˌɪrɪˈspektɪv/ — *adj*. in spite of everything 无关的;不考虑的;不顾的

victory /ˈvɪkt(ə)rɪ/ — *n*. a successful ending of a struggle or contest 胜利;成功

defeat /dɪˈfiːt/ — *n*. an unsuccessful ending to a struggle or contest 失败
vt. to win a victory over 击败;战胜;挫败

interact /ˌɪntərˈækt/ — *v*. to act together or towards others or with others 互相影响;互相作用

collaborate /kəˈlæbəreɪt/ — *vi*. to work together on a common enterprise of project 合作;协作

harness /ˈhɑːnɪs/ — *vt*. ① to exploit the power of 利用 ② to control and direct with or as if by reins 治理;驾驭 ③ to put a harness 披上甲胄
n. stable gear consisting of an arrangement of leather straps fitted to a draft animal so that it can be attached to and pull a cart 马具;甲胄

delegation /ˌdelɪˈgeɪʃ(ə)n/ — *n*. ① a group of representatives or delegates 代表团 ② authorizing subordinates to make certain decisions 授权;委托

confidence /ˈkɒnfɪd(ə)ns/ — *n*. freedom from doubt;belief in yourself and your abilities 信心;信任

accomplishment /əˈkʌmplɪʃm(ə)nt/ — *n*. the action of accomplishing something 成就;完成

bounce /baʊns/ — *n*. the quality of a substance that is able to rebound 跳;弹力
v. to spring back;to spring away from an impact 弹跳;弹起;反跳;弹回

clap /klæp/ — *v*. to hit one's hands or shout after performances to indicate approval 鼓掌,拍手
n. a sudden very loud noise 鼓掌;拍手声

endorphin /enˈdɔːfɪn/ — *n*. a neurochemical occurring naturally in the brain and having analgesic properties 脑内啡

bust /bʌst/ — *v*. ① to ruin completely 破坏;爆裂 ② to go bankrupt 破产
n. ① a complete failure 失败 ② chest 胸部

cholesterol /kəˈlestərɒl/ — *n*. an animal sterol that is normally synthesized by the liver; the most abundant steroid in animal tissues 胆固醇

diabetes /ˌdaɪəˈbiːtiːz/ — *n*. any of several metabolic disorders marked by excessive urination and persistent thirst 糖尿病;多尿症

hypertension /ˌhaɪpəˈtenʃ(ə)n/ — *n*. a common disorder in which blood pressure remains abnormally high (a reading of 140/90 mm Hg or greater) 高血压

disorder /dɪsˈɔːdə/ — *n*. condition in which there is a disturbance of normal functioning 混乱;骚乱

strain /streɪn/ — *n*. difficulty that causes worry or emotional tension 压力;负担
v. to exert much effort or energy 拉紧;尽力

depression /dɪˈpreʃ(ə)n/ — *n*. ① a mental state characterized by a pessimistic sense of inadequacy and a despondent lack of activity 沮丧 ② a long-term economic state characterized by unemployment and low prices and low levels of trade and investment 不景气;萧条

psychological /ˌsaɪkəˈlɒdʒɪk(ə)l/   *adj*. of or relating to or determined by psychology 心理的;心理学的;精神上的

achieve /əˈtʃiːv/   *v*. to gain with effort 取得;获得;实现;成功

combination /ˌkɒmbɪˈneɪʃ(ə)n/   *n*. a collection of things that have been combined; an assemblage of separate parts or qualities 结合;组合;联合

recreation /ˌrekrɪˈeɪʃ(ə)n/   *n*. an activity that diverts or amuses or stimulates 娱乐;消遣;休养

advantageous /ˌædvənˈteɪdʒəs/   *adj*. giving an advantage 有利的;有益的

invest /ɪnˈvest/   *vt*. & *vi*. to make an investment 投资;入股

Phrases and Expressions

serve as	担任……;充当……;起……的作用
put to good use	充分利用
engage in	从事于;参加
expose to	暴露于;使处于……的影响之下
irrespective of	不顾的;不考虑的;无论
interact with	与……相互作用
give sb. the high	让……开心
at a risk of	冒……风险
deal with	处理;涉及;做生意
be prone to	易于……;有……的倾向
invest in	投资于;买进;寄希望于

Text Notes

1. 此句中 playing some sport 和 maintaining your physical and mental well-being 两个现在分词短语分别作句子主语和介词 in 的宾语,go a long way 意为"对……大有帮助"。例如:The findings suggest that good control of blood sugar, blood pressure and cholesterol can go a long way toward preventing or slowing diabetic eye disease. 研究结果表明,对血糖、血压和血脂进行有效的控制对于预防和减缓糖尿病性眼病有很大的帮助。本句的意思是:有规律地参加体育运动对于保持生理和心理健康很有帮助。

2. put sth. to good use 意为"充分利用"。例如:Much of our refuse could actually be put to good use if the efficient garbage treatment systems were available. 如果采用有效的垃圾处理系统,大部分垃圾实际上可以得到很好的利用。本句中 put to good use 为过去分词修饰先行词 energy。

3. irrespective of 为介词短语,意为"不考虑的""不管"。例如:We have to leave today irrespective of the harsh weather. 不管天气有多糟糕,我们今天必须出发。whether 所引导的句子为宾语从句,做介词 of 的宾语。本句的意思是:不管结果是胜利还是失败,运动总能够培养孩子的竞争意识及参与意识。

4. which 引导的是一个定语从句,修饰先行词 exercise。现在分词短语 thus restoring your mental health 为结果状语。本句的意思是:换言之,运动是一种锻炼方式,能够在你体内产生快乐分子,从而使你恢复精神健康。

5. 此句中 as 引导的是原因状语从句,it won't come as a surprise ... 是主句。It 为主句的形式主语,并无实际语义,只是为满足语法上的需要,避免句子头重脚轻,它替代的是句子的逻辑主语,即that 引导的句子。本句的意思是:由于运动是一种完美的锻炼形式,它有诸如降低血压,维持血糖和胆固醇正常水平,减少其他健康隐患等健康益处也就不足为奇了。

Text Comprehension

Please choose the best answers to the following questions according to the text.

1. Which of the following statements about sports is wrong?
   A. Sports are kinds of physical exercise.
   B. Sports have nothing to do with Math skills in children.
   C. Sports make us happy.
   D. Sports are beneficial to the development of social skills.

2. How do sports make people happy?
   A. By increasing endorphins in the brain.
   B. By making people physically exhausted.
   C. By getting more people involved in exercises.
   D. By allowing people to be the winner of life.

3. What does the phrase "engaging in" mean in Para. 2?
   A. Taking part in.   B. Communicating with.
   C. Falling in love with.   D. Resulting in.

4. Sports offer people the following health benefits except _____.
   A. lowering blood pressure   B. maintaining blood sugar
   C. reducing many health risks   D. making people sleep well

5. How many sports are mentioned to help children increase focus?
   A. 2   B. 4   C. 6   D. 8

Vocabulary and Structure

Please choose the best answer for each of the following sentences.

1. And that is really the problem, irrespective _____ what this site turns out to be.
   A. to   B. of
   C. in   D. with

2. It can _____ the go-between for your personal and career schedules.
   A. stand up   B. participate in
   C. serve as   D. put to

3. Jack won the championship of the competition, _____ made the whole family excited.
   A. that   B. who
   C. which   D. what

4. The aim is neither to judge nor to force forgiveness, but rather to _____ understanding.
   A. foster   B. harvest
   C. brighten   D. activate

5. Patients with the condition are _____ a higher risk of a number of complications.
   A. in   B. on   C. at   D. with

Comprehensive Exercise

There are five incomplete sentences in the following passage. Read the passage and choose the word that best fits into the passage. Do remember each word can be used only once.

A. to   B. origin   C. own   D. popular   E. numbers

Every sport has its own history of __1__, and obviously has also come a long way since the time it was first played. With the number of sports played all around the world today, and the arrival of satellite television, these sports are also followed and watched in large __2__ by people all around the globe. Hence, arises the debate as __3__ which are the most popular sports in the world. Everyone has their __4__ favorites, and some sports are more __5__ in different parts of the world. But there are a few that are followed worldwide, and have an unbelievable fan base.

Translation

Please translate the following sentences into Chinese.

1. Education is the best way for a nation to invest in the future.
2. Any size of donation would be very much appreciated and put to good use.
3. Dispose of batteries properly. Do not throw them into fire or expose to high temperature.
4. Even if we achieve great success in our work, we should not be conceited.
5. What they lack is a sense of how people share and collaborate.

■■ Text B   Father's Eyes

Anonymous

Bob Richards, the former pole-vault champion, shares a moving story about a skinny young boy who loved football with all his heart.[1] Practice after practice, he eagerly gave everything he had. But being half the size of the other boys[2], he got absolutely nowhere. At all the games, this hopeful athlete sat on the bench and hardly ever played.

This teenager lived alone with his father, and the two of them had a very special relationship. Even though the son was always on the bench, his father was always in the stands cheering. He never missed a game.

The young man was determined to try his best at every practice, and perhaps he'd get to play when he became a senior. All through high school he never missed a practice nor a game but remained a bench-warmer all four years.

His faithful father was always in the stands, always with words of encouragement for him.

When the young man went to college, he decided to try out for the football team as a "walk-on". Everyone was sure he could never make the cut, but he did. The coach admitted that he kept him on the roster because he always put his heart and soul to every practice, and at the same time, provided the other members with the spirit and hustle they badly needed.[3]

It was the end of his senior football season, and as he trotted onto the practice field shortly before the big playoff game, the coach met him with a telegram.

The young man read the telegram and he became deathly silent. Swallowing hard, he mumbled to the coach, "my father died this morning. Is it all right if I miss practice today?" The coach put his arm gently around his shoulder[4] and said, "Take the rest of the week off, son. And don't even plan to come back to the game on Saturday."

Saturday arrived, and the game was not going well. In the third quarter, when the team was ten points behind, a silent young man quietly slipped into the empty locker room and put on his football gear. As he ran onto the sidelines, the coach and his players were astounded to see their faithful teammate back so soon. "Coach, please let me play. I've just got to play today," said the young man. The coach pretended not to hear him. There was no way he wanted his worst player in this close playoff game. But the young man persisted, and finally feeling sorry for the kid, the coach gave in. "All right," he said. "You can go in."

Before long, the coach, the players and everyone in the stands could not believe their eyes. This little unknown, who had never played before, was doing everything right. The opposing team could not stop him. He ran, passed, blocked, and tackled like a star. His team began to triumph. The score was soon tied. In the closing seconds of the game, this kid intercepted a pass and ran all the way for the winning touchdown.

Finally, after the stands had emptied and the team had showered and left the locker room, the coach noticed that this young man was sitting quietly in the corner all alone. The coach came to him and said, "kid, I can't believe it. You were fantastic! Tell me what got into you? How did you do it?"

He looked at the coach, with tears in his eyes, and said, "well, you knew my dad died, but did you know that my dad was blind?" The young man swallowed hard[5] and forced a smile, "dad came to all my games, but today was the first time he could see me play, and I wanted to show him I could do it."

New Words

former /ˈfɔːmə/	*adj.* referring to the first of two things or persons mentioned 从前的;前者的
pole-vault /ˈpəʊlvɔːlt/	*n.* a competition that involves jumping over a high crossbar with the aid of a long pole 撑竿跳
champion /ˈtʃæmpɪən/	*n.* someone who has won first place in a competition 冠军
skinny /ˈskɪnɪ/	*adj.* being very thin 皮的;皮包骨的
eagerly /ˈiːgəlɪ/	*adv.* with eagerness; in an eager manner 急切地;渴望地;热心地
absolutely /ˈæbsəluːtlɪ/	*adv.* totally and definitely; without question 绝对地;完全地
hopeful /ˈhəʊpfʊl/	*adj.* having or manifesting or inspiring hope 有希望的;有前途的
athlete /ˈæθliːt/	*n.* a person trained to compete in sports 运动员;体育家

teenager /'ti:neɪdʒə/   *n*. a juvenile between the onset of puberty and maturity 十几岁的青少年；十三岁到十九岁的少年

relationship /rɪˈleɪʃ(ə)nʃɪp/   *n*. a relation between people 关系；关联

stand /stænd/   *n*. ① tiered seats consisting of a structure where people can sit to watch an event 看台 ② the position where a thing or person stands 立场

bench /ben(t)ʃ/   *n*. ① a long seat for more than one person 长凳 ② the reserve players on a team 替补队员

senior /'si:nɪə/   *adj*. ① older 年长的 ② higher in rank 地位较高的；高级的 ③ longer in length of tenure or service 资格较老的
   n. a person who is older than you are 上司；较年长者

bench-warmer /'bentʃˌwɔːmə/   *n*. (sports) a substitute who seldom plays 候补球员

faithful /'feɪθfʊl/   *adj*. steadfast in affection or allegiance 忠实的；忠诚的；如实的；准确可靠的

walk-on /'wɔːkɒn/   *n*. someone who plays a small part in a dramatic production or sports 跑龙套角色；临时队员

roster /'rɒstə/   *n*. a list of names 花名册；执勤人员表

hustle /'hʌs(ə)l/   *v*. to move or cause to move energetically or busily 催促；猛推
   n. a rapid active commotion 推；奔忙；拥挤喧嚷

trot /trɒt/   *v*. to run at a moderately swift pace 小跑；慢跑；快步走
   n. a slow pace of running 慢跑

shortly /'ʃɔːtlɪ/   *adv*. for a short time 立刻；简短地

deathly /'deθlɪ/   *adv. & adj*. in the manner of death 死一般的；致命的；死了一样地

swallow /'swɒləʊ/   *v*. to pass through the esophagus as part of eating or drinking 吞下；咽下
   n. ① the act of swallowing 吞咽；一次吞咽的量 ② small long-winged songbird noted for swift graceful flight and the regularity of its migrations 燕子

mumble /'mʌmb(ə)l/   *v*. to talk indistinctly, usually in a low voice 含糊地说
   n. a soft indistinct utterance 含糊的话；咕噜

coach /kəʊtʃ/   *n*. ① (sports) someone in charge of training an athlete or a team 教练 ② a vehicle carrying many passengers used for public transport 长途公车
   v. to teach and supervise 训练；指导

quarter /'kwɔːtə/   *n*. ① one of four equal parts 四分之一 ② a unit of time equal to 15 minutes or a quarter of an hour 一刻钟 ③ one fourth of match time 四分之一场

slip /slɪp/   *v*. ① to move stealthily 滑动 ② to make a mistake 犯错 ③ to insert inconspicuously or quickly or quietly 塞入；溜入
   n. ① a slippery smoothness 滑；溜 ② mistake 错误

sideline /'saɪdlaɪn/   *n*. a line that marks the side boundary of a playing field 球场边线
   vt. to remove from the center of activity or attention; to place

into an inferior position 迫使退出

astound /əˈstaʊnd/	*vt.* to affect with wonder 使惊骇;使震惊
teammate /ˈtiːmmeɪt/	*n.* a fellow member of a team 队友;同队队员
pretend /prɪˈtend/	*vt.* to make believe with the intent to deceive 假装;伪装;佯装
playoff /ˈpleɪˌɒf/	*n.* any final competition to determine a championship 双方得分相等时的最后决赛;复赛;季后赛
persist /pəˈsɪst/	*v.* to be persistent; to refuse to stop 坚持;持续
block /blɒk/	*v.* to hinder or to prevent the progress or accomplishment 阻止;阻塞;限制 *n.* ① a solid piece of something (usually having flat rectangular sides) 块 ② a rectangular area in a city surrounded by streets and usually containing several buildings 街区
tackle /ˈtæk(ə)l/	*vt. & vi.* ① to seize and throw down an opponent player, who usually carries the ball 拦截抢球 ② to deal with 处理 ③ to take hold of 抓住
intercept /ˌɪntəˈsept/	*v.* to seize on its way 拦截;截断
touchdown /ˈtʌtʃdaʊn/	*n.* being in possession of the ball across the opponents' goal line 触地;触地得分
shower /ˈʃaʊə/	*n.* ① washing yourself by standing upright under water sprayed from a nozzle 淋浴 ② a sudden downpour 一阵;阵雨 *v.* ①to take a shower 淋浴 ② to rain abundantly 下阵雨
locker /ˈlɒkə/	*n.* a storage compartment for clothes and valuables usually with a lock 有锁的存物柜
fantastic /fænˈtæstɪk/	*adj.* ① extraordinarily good 极好的;极出色的 ② existing in fancy only 不可思议的;不切实际的 ③ ludicrously odd 奇异的

Phrases and Expressions

get nowhere	一事无成;无进展
be determined to do	坚决;下决心做……
try one's best	努力;尽力
try out for	竞争;参加选拔
make the cut	达到标准;过关
take one day off	休息一天
slip into	溜入;陷入;渐渐养成
before long	不久以后

Text Notes

1. 此句中 the former pole-vault champion 作为同位语解释 Bob Richards 的身份,即前撑杆跳冠军鲍勃·理查德;who 引导的定语从句修饰先行词 young boy。

2. being half the size of the other boys 意为"其他男孩子体型的一半",get nowhere 意为"毫无进展"

"一事无成"。例如：The negotiation got nowhere. 谈判毫无进展。

3. put one's heart and soul to do sth. 意为"全身心地投入去做某事"。例如：Sometimes it is too hard to put your heart and soul to do one thing. 有时候让自己全身心地投入做一件事太难了。provide sb. with sth. 意为"向某人提供某物"。例如：Please provide us with any example of your previous job. 请提供您任一工作案例。此句中 because 引导的原因状语从句中有两个谓语动词，分别为 put 和 provide。本句的意思是：不仅因为他总是全身心地投入练习，也是因为他展现了其他球员迫切需要的坚强和斗志。

4. put one's arm around one's shoulder 意为"搂住某人的肩膀"，take the rest of the week off 意为"这周余下的日子休息"。例如：I want to take one day off. 我想休息一天。

5. swallow hard 意为"用力吞了下口水"，force a smile 意为"强挤出点笑容"。

Text Comprehension

Please read the following statements and mark T/F according to the text.

1. The young boy lived with his parents.
   A. T   B. F
2. The coach accepted the young boy because he was wretched.
   A. T   B. F
3. The young boy's father was a deaf.
   A. T   B. F
4. The young boy never missed practice even if his father died.
   A. T   B. F
5. The young boy succeeded in proving himself in the end.
   A. T   B. F

Vocabulary and Structure

Please complete the following sentences with the proper forms of the words given.

1. My boss told me that what finally won her over was my _____ . (persist)
2. He will be able to take up his normal routine _____ . (short)
3. I dialed the combination to open my _____ . (lock)
4. The _____ girl was still trying to lose more weight. (skin)
5. He didn't _____ his homework until nine o'clock. (tackled)

Translation

Please translate the following passage into Chinese.

Being half the size of the other boys, he got absolutely nowhere. The young man was determined to try his best at every practice, and perhaps he'd get to play when he became a senior. He ran, passed, blocked, and tackled like a star. His team began to triumph. In the closing seconds of the game, this kid intercepted a pass and ran all the way for the winning touchdown.

Further Study

（Apologies）

Communication Skills

道歉（Apologies）：道歉是社交中常见而重要的一环。要注意道歉需诚恳有礼貌。

Key Sentences

◆ Making apologies
○ I am terribly/awfully sorry for . . . .
○ Sorry, I didn't mean it.
○ Please forgive me for my rudeness.
○ How could I be so thoughtless as to make such a mistake?
○ I am sorry. I do apologize about/for all the trouble.
◆ Responding to apologies
○ Forget it.
○ Never mind.
○ It is not your fault.
○ You really don't have to worry about it.
○ There is no need for you to worry.

Practice

1. — I am afraid I spilled coffee on the tablecloth.

   — _____

   A. Don't worry about it.   B. What's wrong with you?
   C. What's happened?   D. You have done well.

2. — I am very sorry. Can I get you another one?

   — _____

   A. That's fine.   B. I don't forgive you.
   C. No, forget about it.   D. It's none of your business.

3. — _____, but I seem to have misplaced your scarf.
   — Oh, that's all right.
   A. I am fine   B. I am sorry   C. It's nice of you   D. I am OK

4. — I must apologize for having delayed the job.

   — _____

   A. Pleased to meet you.   B. No, that's not your fault.
   C. I don't know.   D. Thanks a lot.

5. — I'm very sorry for the mistake I've made.

— It's OK. _____

A. That can happen to the rest of us.   B. What's the matter with you?

C. Why are you so careless?   D. You should be responsible for it.

Grammar

双宾语 (double objects)：在英语中，有些及物动词可接两个宾语（双宾语），即指人的间接宾语和指物的直接宾语。

常用句型为：主语 + 及物动词 + 间接宾语 + 直接宾语。

例如：She gave me a cup of tea. 她给了我一杯茶。

有时，间接宾语也可改为由介词 to 或 for 引导的短语，放在直接宾语的后面。

例如：She passed him the salt. = She passed the salt to him. 她把盐递给了他。

注：由 to 连接间接宾语的动词有：pass, give, show, tell, lend, take 等；由 for 连接间接宾语的动词有：buy, cook, get, sing, make 等。

例如：On the bus, he often gives his seat to an old person. 在公共汽车上，他经常把座位让给老人。

例如：Mother cooks breakfast for us every day. 母亲每天都为我们做早饭。

宾语补足语 (object complement)：在英语中，有些动词除了一个宾语外，还需要一个成分来补充说明宾语的情况，这样句子意义才能表达完整。这种成分在英语中被称为宾语补足语（或叫复合宾语）。

这类常用的动词有：make, have, get, let, see, consider, find, cause, help 等。

例如：May I help you plant the tree? 我能帮你种树吗？

宾语补足语的几种类型：

一、名词（包括名词性物主代词）作宾语补足语

例如：I can't understand why people elected her monitor. 我不明白人们为什么选她当班长。

二、形容词及其短语作宾语补足语

例如：Please keep the windows open. We need more fresh air. 请让窗户开着，我们需要更多的新鲜空气。

三、不定式短语作宾语补足语

常接带 to 的动词不定式作宾语补足语的动词有：ask, tell, want, teach, wish 等。

例如：I often ask him to help me with my English. 我经常请他帮助我学习英语。

注：下列动词后的不定式作宾补时省略 to：see, watch, hear, make, let, have。

例如：I can't have you say so. 我不能让你这么说。

例如：You should try your best to make him understand that. 你应该尽量让他明白那件事。

四、现在分词短语作宾语补足语

跟现在分词作宾语补足语的动词有：catch, have, get, keep, hear, find, feel, leave, make 等。

例如：I caught her stealing in the bookshop. 我当场抓住她在书店行窃。

五、过去分词短语作宾语补足语

例如：When they got there，they found the bank robbed. 当他们到那儿的时候，就发现银行被抢了。

不定式作宾语补足语表示动作的过程，现在分词作宾语补足语表示宾语正在进行的动作，过去分词作宾语补足语表示动作的完成，有时含有被动意义。

六、介词短语作宾语补足语

例如：Please make yourself at home. 请随意。

七、副词作宾语补足语

例如：He ordered them away. 他命令他们离开。

八、从句作宾语补足语

例如：We will soon make our school what your school is now. 我们很快会把我们学校变成你校那样。

Practice

1. I am tired. Would you like to fetch a chair _____ me?
   A. in　　　　　　　B. for　　　　　　　C. at　　　　　　　D. of

2. Though he had often made his little sister _____ , today he was made _____ by his little sister.
   A. cry；to cry　　　　　　　B. crying；crying
   C. cry；cry　　　　　　　　D. to cry；cry

3. The manager discussed the plan that they would like to see _____ the next year.
   A. carry out　　　　　　　B. carrying out
   C. carried out　　　　　　D. to carry out

4. They would not allow him _____ across the enemy line.
   A. to risk going　　　　　　B. risking to go
   C. for risk to go　　　　　　D. risk going

5. With a lot of difficult problems _____ , the newly-elected president is having a hard time.
   A. settled　　　　B. settling　　　　C. to settle　　　　D. being settled

Writing

拒绝信（Letter of Rejection）：就所收到的邀请告知对方自己因为某些原因而不能接受的信件。书写此类信件时，措辞一定要礼貌含蓄，所有信息点皆须囊括在内。

拒绝信一般包括以下三个部分：

首先，在拒绝信中，写作的前提就是自己已经接到了别人的邀请，并对别人的邀请表示感谢。其次，才要表明目的，告知对方自己不能接受，并简要陈述理由。句子必须礼貌真挚，用语一定要委婉。

例如：It gives me great pleasure to be invited to attend ... I would like to accept your warm invitation but I cannot due to an earlier appointment.

其次，就是要向对方解释自己不能接受邀请的具体原因。需要记住的是要逻辑严谨。

例如：Two weeks ago, I made an appointment with one of my former colleagues

最后，紧接前面内容，向对方解释完原因之后，就要为自己不能接受邀请而进行道歉了。同时，虽然不能亲自应邀前往，但是也要表达美好祝愿，这也是人际交流的常识与礼貌。

例如：Therefore, I feel terribly sorry for being unable to attend the event. I wish the ceremony a success.

Practice

Instruction：假如你叫王雷，昨天收到你的学生麦克的一封信邀请你参加他的毕业典礼。请写一封回绝信，告知你无法前往，陈述理由并表示歉意。

Unit Three
Manners

Guidance

1. This unit consists of Text A, Text B and Further Study. **Text A** tells us how good manners are appreciated as much as bad manners are abhorred. **Text B** introduces etiquettes of graduation ceremony and provides some suggestions on how to prepare for the ceremony. **Further Study** focuses on communication skills.

2. By learning this unit, students will be able to master the structure of the texts, new words, phrases and expressions. Students will improve their understanding of grammatical structures, reading comprehension and enlarge their vocabulary by doing the relevant exercises. Meanwhile, they will gain better understanding on *Manners*.

3. **Further study** aims to improve students' skills for communication. By doing the exercises, students will know how to ask for information. They will also learn knowledge on object clause and how to write a narration.

- Basic Table Manners
- Etiquettes of Graduation Ceremony

> Good manners will open doors that the best education cannot.
>
> — Clarence Thomas

▪▪ Text A　Basic Table Manners

Lisa Plancich[1]

The good looks of a man and his manners are two different things. A man might have

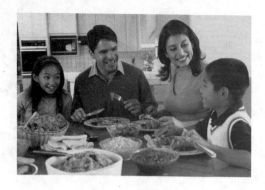

good looks, but he becomes attractive and beautiful only if[2] he has pleasing manners and good deeds. Our actions and manners are noticed by all. Manners are the ornaments that make a woman a lady and a man a gentleman.

Lunching in a restaurant, the gentlemen at my table immediately noticed three rather pretty women who entered and were seated near our table. All three women were quite striking and very well dressed. Their hair was neat and I was impressed with their choice in shoes and bags. Seated at the table next to these young women were four other women all dressed much more conservatively. Although they were professional looking, they were not what the men at my table considered show stoppers.[3]

The ladies at the "pretty table" sat down heavily, as though they were dealing with a tiring day. One told the server they wanted water with lemon and asked him to bring them straws. The only reason I remember what was said is all three were very loud.[4] Suddenly one burped, also loud, and everyone at their table laughed. One of them snorted when they laughed and the giggles started all over again. This time it was followed by four letter words[5] by one of the three commenting on how gross they were being.

When their server arrived with the water all three ladies were very rude. They all had special requests and acted as though they had already decided that their server or the chefs were going to mess up their requests.

Meanwhile at the more business-like table, I noticed smiles and laughter. They were quite kind to the same server who had endured rudeness earlier.

Drinks at the pretty table resulted in sugar in an iced tea followed by the noisiest spoon swirling the sugar I have ever endured. Another slurped her tea. The third complained that she was sure she was drinking Coke and not Pepsi. No one thanked the server for bringing their drinks. No one smiled. All three had their elbows on the table, chin in their hands.

At the business table all four thanked their server for their drinks. No one clinked a spoon. No one was rude. All three smiled. Suddenly these more business-like women became the most beautiful people in the restaurant.

A change was definitely occurring. Clearly first impressions are not always true. At the pretty table, manners deteriorated to nonexistence. There were mouths full of food and entire conversations going on simultaneously. Elbows supported chins. No napkins were used. It was a sad sight.

The business table was the model of good manners. Laughter was gentle. Napkins were used. Conversation was quick but no one had food in their mouth when they spoke. The difference between the two tables was extreme. By the time the gentlemen and I had left, no one gave the formerly pretty women a second glance. Without their realizing it, what was cute was now inconsiderate. And what was unnoticed at first became the table who people were attempting to get their attention.

The lunch ended with once striking women deteriorating before our eyes strictly because common courtesy and table manners Mom and Dad taught at a young age were not followed. In the case of making a positive first impression, clearly parents know best.

New Words

burp /bɜːp/
vt. & vi. ① to cause (a baby) to expel gas from the stomach, as by patting the back after feeding 使(婴儿)打嗝 ② to make a noise when air from your stomach passes out through your mouth 打嗝

chef /ʃef/
n. someone who cooks food in a restaurant as their job 厨师;炊事员

chin /tʃɪn/
n. the center of the bottom part of your face, below your mouth and above your neck 颏;下颌

clink /klɪŋk/
vt. & vi. to make or cause to make a light, sharp ringing sound (使)发出玻璃撞击声
n. a light, sharp ringing sound, as of glass or metal 玻璃撞击声

comment /ˈkɒment/
vt. & vi. to make a written or spoken remark, especially giving an opinion 评论;评述
n. a written or spoken remark giving an opinion 点评;评论

conservatively /kənˈsɜːrvətɪvlɪ/
adv. not willing to accept much change, especially in the traditional values of society 保守地;谨慎地

conversation /kɒnvəˈseɪʃn/
n. a talk between two or more people, usually a private and informal one 交谈;谈话;对话

courtesy /ˈkɜːtəsɪ/
n. polite behavior that shows respect for people in social situations 礼貌的行为;周到的举止

cute /kjuːt/
adj. appealing or attractive, usually small esp. in a pretty way 可爱的;惹人喜爱的;小巧精致的

elbow /ˈelbəʊ/
n. the part in the middle of your arm, where it bends 手肘;肘部
vt. & vi. to push or hit someone with your elbow 推挤;用手肘推开

endure /ɪnˈdjʊə/
vt. & vi. ① to suffer something difficult or unpleasant in a patient way over a long period 容忍;忍受 ② to continue in existence;last 耐用;耐久

extreme /ɪkˈstriːm/
adj. being in or attaining the greatest or highest degree;very intense 极度的;极限的

giggle /ˈɡɪɡl/
vt. & vi. to laugh in a nervous, excited, or silly way that is difficult to control 傻笑;咯咯笑

glance /ɡlɑːns/
vi. to look somewhere quickly and then look away 一瞥;看一下
n. a quick look at someone or something 草草地看;浏览

gross /ɡrəʊs/
adj. ① very unpleasant 令人不快的 ② being the total amount of sth. before anything is taken away 总的;毛的

impression /ɪmˈpreʃn/	*n.* the opinion that other people have about you because of the way that you look，speak，or behave 印象；形象
inconsiderate /ˌɪnkənˈsɪdərət/	*adj.* not thinking about other people and their feelings 不体贴的；不考虑他人的
mess /mes/	*n.* ① a situation in which a place is dirty or not neat 脏乱；混乱 ② a difficult situation with a lot of problems，especially because people have made mistakes 困境；窘况；麻烦
napkin /ˈnæpkɪn/	*n.* ① a piece of cloth or paper used for protecting your clothes and wiping your mouth and hands while you are eating 餐巾 ② a sanitary pad 尿布；尿片
ornament /ˈɔːnəmənt/	*vt.* to add something to something else to make it more beautiful 装饰；美化；点缀
	n. a small attractive object used for decoration or for making someone or something more beautiful 装饰品；点缀物
professional /prəˈfeʃnl/	*adj.* relating to work that needs special skills and qualifications 职业的；专职的
	n. someone who has special skills and qualifications 专业人员；专业人士
rudeness /ˈruːdnəs/	*n.* the state of being insulting or uncivil; discourteous; impolite 粗鲁；不礼貌
slurp /slɜːp/	*v.* to eat or drink something noisily 吧唧着吃；发出声音地吃
	n. a loud sucking noise made in eating or drinking 咕噜声；吧唧声
snort /snɔːt/	*n.* a sudden loud noise that you make through your nose，for example because you are angry or laughing 发出哼声；冷笑；轻蔑的大笑
	v. to make a sudden loud noise through your nose，for example because you are angry or laughing 轻蔑的哼声
straw /strɔː/	*n.* ① the yellow stems of dried crops such as wheat 秸秆；禾秆 ② a long thin paper or plastic tube that you use for drinking 吸管
swirl /swɜːl/	*vt. & vi.* to move quickly in circles，or to make something move in this way （使）回旋；（使）打转

Phrases and Expressions

be full of	满的；充满……的
be impressed with	被……所打动；对……留下了深刻的印象
comment on	就……发表看法；对……加以评论
next to	接近……的；跟……邻近的；仅次于……的

Text Notes

1. Lisa Plancich：Etiquette Editor for BellaOnline which was founded in 1999 as a web site for continuously fresh content in many categories to represent "The Voice of Women on the Web".

2. only if 意为"仅仅如果",用于引导条件状语从句。if only 用于虚拟语气,表示"要是……就好了"。例如:If only one had an unlimited supply of money! 要是财源不断就好了!(与现在事实相反)

3. 此句为倒装句,表语 Seated at the table next to these young women 前置起到强调的作用。此句可翻译为:就在这些年轻女子旁边的桌子,坐着四位女士,她们穿着都非常保守。"Show stoppers" means something that is strikingly attractive or has great popular appeal. 即:吸引人的人或事。

4. the reason 意为"原因是",此处省略了关系代词 that,that 后是定语从句,整句可译为:我记得她们说了什么的原因是她们谈话的声音非常大。

5. four letter words 意为"粗俗的下流话"。英语中所谓的 four-letter words 其实可以翻译为"四字母粗俗词",因其常由四个字母组成,故名。此类词多与性及排泄有关,如 piss, shit 等等。

Text Comprehension

Please choose the best answers to the following questions according to the text.

1. What's the article's general idea?
   A. People should not make much noise while eating in a restaurant.
   B. People should be well dressed when eating in a restaurant.
   C. People should obey some certain table manners when eating in a restaurant.
   D. Beautiful women are welcomed everywhere.

2. Why did the professional looking women not catch the author and her friends' attention?
   A. Because the professional looking women sit far away from them.
   B. Because the author and her friends did not want to pay attention to anyone.
   C. Because their appearance were not attractive.
   D. Because they were old.

3. Which statement is true according to the article?
   A. The women in the "pretty table" were rude to the waiter.
   B. The author could hear the talk of women at the "pretty table" because they sat close.
   C. The women at the "pretty table" worked hard during the daytime.
   D. One of the women in the "pretty table" kept silent.

4. Why did the professional women get people's attention at last?
   A. Because they changed their clothes and put on makeup.
   B. Because people found out who they really were.
   C. Because their behavior were elegant.
   D. Because they smiled at everyone.

5. Which of the following behaviors is not necessary to achieve good manners?
   A. Never talk with your mouth full.
   B. Use napkins when eating.
   C. Always wear makeup when dating with friends.
   D. Talk in low voice in public.

Vocabulary and Structure

Please choose the best answer for each of the following sentences.

1. _____ at the meeting are some experienced teachers.
   A．Presented   B．Having been present
   C．Being presented   D．Present

2. You can make progress _____ you are modest.
   A．only if   B．if only
   C．because of   D．on that

3. _____ from the hill，our school looks more beautiful.
   A．Seeing   B．Seen
   C．Being seen   D．Saw

4. While I was working for that company，I had to _____ consumer affairs.
   A．deal on   B．deal in
   C．deal with   D．deal for

5. The expert made an impersonal comment _____ the incident.
   A．with   B．to
   C．in   D．on

Comprehensive Exercise

There are five incomplete sentences in the following passage. Read the passage and choose the word that best fits into the passage. Do remember each word can be used only once.

A．therefore   B．finally   C．up   D．defined   E．on

Etiquettes simply mean good manners. Don't mess __1__ your interview by being brash. Follow these simple etiquette tips to come across as a well-groomed and perfect candidate.

So，__2__ your resume has landed you a job interview. This is your first opportunity to make a lasting impression __3__ the organization of your dreams. When your interview begins，however，job sills become secondary. What matters more now is the kind of person you are. Your manners — good or bad will show them who you really are.

Etiquette can be __4__ simply as the grand set of all good manners. Etiquette is a language used to relate your respect and consideration to others. __5__ , the day of your interview is not the time to appear unprofessional，disrespectful of inconsiderate by violating any of the following etiquette tips.

Translation

Please translate the following sentences into Chinese.

1. I was very impressed by the waiter's great courtesy in the five-star hotel.
2. The spoon is right next to the fork.
3. He talks as though he were a teacher.

4. The only reason I was late is my car had broken down.

5. Manners are the ornaments that make a woman a lady and a man a gentleman.

■■ Text B Etiquettes of Graduation Ceremony

Anonymous

According to the 2013 World Happiness Report, America is considered the 17th happiest country in the world. However, America is one of the few nations with freedom, equal rights and wealth. Why aren't we happier?

Every student dreams of walking across the stage wearing a graduation cap & gown and receive a graduation diploma or certificate from the professors. Every student in each college and university looks forward to doing this. They work hard to be eligible for the graduation diploma. And finally, the day comes and their dream comes true. Happiness and sense of achievement is all what the students want to experience on this important day. Wearing a graduation cap and gown is a tradition in graduation ceremony. As a result, caps and gowns for graduation are considered as the symbol of achievement and viewed with respect. So, it's the duty of every student to follow this etiquette during the graduation ceremony.

First of all you have to get a perfect cap and gown before the graduation ceremony. They can be got from the university or a local store. Find out what ways you have in order to save some money. You can try buying or renting the complete robe from a store that offers discounts. Do enquire about the colour and style that your university has set up. It will look abnormal if you attend graduation ceremony wearing different coloured caps & gowns that your school does not follow. This is definitely not a way to stand out of the crowd.

Before you become a part of the grand event of graduation, you should practice wearing your graduation cap. Wear it in such a way that the tassel hanging from the cap won't obstruct your vision. The more you wear the cap, the more you will be comfortable wearing it for long time. [1] Again, as you become more familiar with the cap, it will not distract you while walking on the stage. [2] You will certainly not wish to walk on the stage as if you are balancing a big bundle of books on your head. The tassel should always hang from the right side of the cap. It doesn't look appropriate if the tassel remains on the front or back or even on the left side of the cap. So adjust the cap accordingly.

When your name is called up, you may feel like dancing. Some students actually start jumping[3] once they are called upon the stage to receive their certificate. However, you should remember that you are wearing a gown and it is likely to tumble while walking in a gown. Hence, one should always practice walking while wearing the gown. When you reach the stage, walk confidently towards principal and receive your certificate. After that, shake hands with the principal. Once you receive the diploma, shift the tassel to the left side of your cap and then go back to your seat. After coming back to your seat, you will have to leave the tassel to left of the cap for the rest of the graduation ceremony.

New Words

abnormal /æb'nɔːml/   *adj*. not usual or typical，especially in a way that is worrying or that shows there may be something wrong or harmful 反常的；异常的

accordingly /ə'kɔːdɪŋlɪ/   *adv*. ① as a result of something 因此；所以；于是 ② in a way that is appropriate to the situation 相应地

achievement /ə'tʃiːvmənt/   *n*. ① the act of accomplishing or finishing 完成；达到；实现 ② something accomplished successfully，especially by means of exertion，skill，practice，or perseverance 成就；成绩

adjust /ə'dʒʌst/   *vt*. & *vi*. ① to change something slightly in order to make it better，more accurate，or more effective 调节；调整 ② to get used to a new situation by changing your ideas or the way you do things 调整(自己)以适应；(使自己)变得适合

appropriate /ə'prəʊprɪət/   *adj*. suitable or right for a particular situation or purpose 适合的；恰当的；妥当的

   vt. ① to decide officially that money will be used for a particular purpose 拨给；拨出 ② to take something for yourself 挪用；盗取

balance /'bæləns/   *n*. ① the ability to remain steady in an upright position 平衡力 ② a situation in which different aspects or features are treated equally or exist in the correct relationship to each other 平衡；均势

   vt. ① to keep your body steady without falling over 保持身体平衡 ② to create or preserve a good or correct balance between different features or aspects 协调；使平衡；使均衡

bundle /'bʌndl/   *n*. a group of things that have been tied together，especially so that you can carry them easily 捆；束；包

ceremony /'serəmənɪ/   *n*. a formal public event with special traditions，actions，or words 仪式；典礼

certificate /sə'tɪfɪkət/   *n*. an official document stating that you have passed an examination，successfully completed a course，or achieved the necessary qualifications to work in a particular profession 证书；凭证

diploma /dɪ'pləʊmə/   *n*. an official document that proves you have successfully finished all the work in a course of study 文凭；学位证书

discount /'dɪskaʊnt/   *n*. a reduction in the price of something 折扣额

   vt. to reduce the price of something 减价；打折

distract /dɪ'strækt/   *vt*. to get someone's attention and prevent them from concentrating on something 使分心；使分散注意力

eligible /'elɪdʒəbl/   *adj*. allowed by rules or laws to do something or to receive something 有资格的;合格的

enquire /ɪnˈkwaɪə/	*vt*. ① to seek information by questioning; ask 询问;打听 ② to make investigation 调查;查究
etiquette /ˈetɪket/	*n*. a set of rules for behaving correctly in social situations 礼仪;礼节
gown /gaʊn/	*n*. ① a special long dress worn by a woman, often for dancing or other special occasions 女士礼服 ② a piece of formal clothing like a loose coat worn by judges and by teachers and students at some ceremonies at schools 礼服;长袍
graduation /ˌgrædʒuˈeɪʃn/	*n*. the act of receiving a diploma or degree after finishing a course of study at a school such as a high school, college, or university 毕业
obstruct /əbˈstrʌkt/	*vt*. ① to block a path, passage, door, etc. so that it is difficult or impossible for someone or something to move along or through it 阻挡;堵塞;使……不通 ② to take action in order to prevent someone from doing something or to prevent something from happening 妨碍;阻碍
principal /ˈprɪnsəpl/	*n*. one who holds a position of presiding rank, especially the head of an elementary school or high school 校长
	adj. first, highest, or foremost in importance, rank, worth, or degree; chief 主要的;首要的;最重要的
procedure /prəˈsiːdʒə/	*n*. a way of doing something, especially the correct or usual way 过程;步骤
professor /prəˈfesə/	*n*. a senior teacher in a college or university 专家;教授
shift /ʃɪft/	*v*. ① to move your body or a part of your body slightly, for example because you are bored 轻微移动;稍微挪动 ② to change 改变;变换
	n. ① a period of work time in a factory, hospital, or other place where some people work during the day and some work at night 班次;工时 ② a change in something, for example in someone's ideas or opinions 改变;变换
symbol /ˈsɪmbl/	*n*. ① someone or something that represents a particular idea or quality 象征;标志 ② a picture or shape used to represent something 符号;记号
tassel /ˈtæsl/	*n*. a group of strings tied together at one end and fastened to clothing or objects as a decoration 穗状物
tumble /ˈtʌmbl/	*n*. an occasion when someone falls to the ground 跌落;摔倒
	vt. & vi. to fall downwards, often hitting the ground several times, but usually without serious injury (使)跌倒;滚落

Phrases and Expressions

be eligible to	合格做某事
be familiar with	对……熟悉
dress up	盛装打扮;特意打扮
look forward to	期待;盼望
set up	安排;准备

Text Notes

1. the more…,the more…句型为"the + 比较级,the + 比较级"结构,常表示"越……,就越……",是一个复合句,其中前面的句子是状语从句,后面的句子是主句。the 用在形容词或副词的比较级前。

2. 以 when,while 引导的时间状语从句和以 if 引导的条件状语从句,谓语动词是主动语态时,如果从句谓语动词所表示的动作是与主句谓语同时发生,可简化为现在分词的一般式。例如:When we heard（= When hearing / Hearing）the teacher's pleasant talk to us, we began to feel comfortable. 当听到老师和我们愉快地谈话时,我们开始自在起来。

3. 像 start,begin,continue,cease 这样一些表示开始,继续和结束意义的动词,既可以接 to do,也可以接 doing,大体上说,意义没有明显的差别。但在某些有限的情况下,start to do sth 意思是指"开始去做某事",有"潜在的可能";start doing sth 意思是指"开始做某事",有"实际进行"的意思。当涉及多次活动时使用 start doing 更为恰当。

Text Comprehension

Please read the following statements and mark T/F according to the text.

1. In most college graduation ceremony, students wear graduation caps and gowns.
   A. T　　　　B. F

2. Students look forward to the graduation ceremony because they think the caps and gowns are very beautiful.
   A. T　　　　B. F

3. The caps and gowns can only be bought in stores.
   A. T　　　　B. F

4. Students can wear gowns in any color as they like.
   A. T　　　　B. F

5. After students get the diploma, the tassel should be shifted to the left side.
   A. T　　　　B. F

Vocabulary and Structure

Please complete the following sentences with the proper forms of the words given

1. Soon after her _____ , she found a job. (graduate)
2. The girl danced on the stage, _____ a pink dress. (wear)
3. All the kids are looking forward to _____ the new teacher. (meet)
4. _____ dumpling on the eve of the spring festival is the tradition for Chinese people. (eat)

5. The more you eat，the _____ you will get.（fat）

Translation

Every student in each college and university looks forward to graduation ceremony. Happiness and sense of achievement is all what the students want to experience on this important day. Wearing a graduation cap and gown is a tradition in graduation ceremony. As a result，caps and gowns for graduation are considered as the symbol of achievement and viewed with respect.

▪▪ Further Study

（**Asking for Information**）

Communication Skills

询问信息（Asking for Information）：询问信息是日常生活中经常遇到的话题，不同的询问内容提问方式也有所不同。

Key Sentences

◆ 问"职业"时用 what ；问"关系"时用 who。例如：
— What is your father?
— He is a doctor.
— Who is that girl?
— She is my classmate（friend / sister）.

◆ 问"品质、外貌、形状、天气情况"等时用 what ... like。例如：
— What is she like ?
— She is honest.
— What is the table like ?
— It is round.
— What's the weather like today?
— It's fine today.

◆ 问"外表看上去怎么样"时用 how。例如：
— How does she look ?
— She looks pretty.
— How do those flowers look?
— They look beautiful.

◆ 问"外貌（表）像谁（什么）"时用 what ... look like。例如：
— What does he look like?
— He looks like our monitor.
— What does this building look like?

— It looks like a tower.

◆ 问"多长时间"时用 how long；问"(在)将来多长时间之后"时用 how soon；问"每隔多长时间"时用 how often。例如：

— How long has he been ill?

— He has been ill for two weeks.

— How soon will he be back?

— He'll be back in two weeks.

— How often do you have your hair cut?

— I have my hair cut once a month.

◆ 问"几月几日"时用 what's the date ...；问"星期几"时用 what day ...。例如：

— What's the date today?

— It's January 15th today.

— What day is it today?

— It's Saturday today.

◆ 问"某物长度"时用 how long；问"距离有多远"时用 how far。例如：

— How long is the bridge?

— It's 800 meters.

— How far is it from your home to your school?

— It's five miles from my home to our school.

Practice

1. — Excuse me，Sir，is the swimming pool open all day?

— _____ . Only from 6：00 pm to 10：00 pm.

   A．That's right   B．Yes, of course

   C．Sorry，I am not sure   D．Sorry，I'm afraid not

2. — I wonder if I could possibly use your car for tonight?

— _____ . I'm not using it anyhow.

   A．Sure，go ahead   B．I don't know

   C．Yes，indeed   D．I don't care

3. — How often do you eat out?

— _____ , but usually once a week.

   A．Have no idea   B．It depends

   C．As usual   D．Generally speaking

4. — Excuse me，could you tell me where I could make a call?

— Sorry，I'm a stranger here.

— _____ .

   A．Thanks a lot   B．That's a pity

   C．Thanks anyway   D．I'm sorry to hear that

5. — Are you satisfied with what she has done?

— _____ . It couldn't be any better.

   A．Not a little   B．Not at all

   C．I'm sorry   D．Thank you

Grammar

宾语从句:在句子中起宾语作用的从句叫做宾语从句。宾语从句分为三类:动词的宾语从句,介词的宾语从句和形容词的宾语从句。宾语从句的结构为:主句 + 连词(引导词) + 宾语从句。

宾语从句构成表:

从句类型	引导词	例句
宾语从句为陈述句	that：that 在从句中不做任何成分,也没有任何具体意思,在口语或非正式场合中常省略	She says（that）she won't take part in the party on Sunday.
宾语从句为一般疑问句	whether 或 if：if/whether 翻译成"是否",具有一定意义,所以不能省略。口语中常用 if	She asked me if/whether she could borrow my books.
宾语从句为特殊疑问句	what, who, whom, which, whose（连接代词）；when, where, how, why（连接副词）：连接代词或连接副词在从句中担任一定的句子成分,具有一定意义,所以不能省略	① Do you know what he said just now? ② I don't remember when we arrived. ③ I asked him where I could get so much money.

Practice

1. Let's see _____ we can find out some information about that city.
   A．that
   B．whether
   C．when
   D．what

2. I have heard _____ he will come tomorrow.
   A．when
   B．how
   C．what
   D．that

3. Could you tell me _____ we are going to meet?
   A．that
   B．whether
   C．who
   D．what

4. Could you tell us _____ gate we have to go to?
   A．that
   B．whether
   C．where
   D．which

5. Could you tell me _____ shall we meet again?
   A．when
   B．that
   C．how
   D．what

Writing

记叙文（Narration）：英语记叙文是记人叙事的文章，它主要是用于说明事件的时间、背景、起因、过程及结果，即我们通常所说的五个"W"（what，who，when，where，why）和一个"H"（how）。记叙文的重点在于"述说"和"描写"，一篇好的记叙文要叙述条理清楚，描写生动形象。因此选材要注意取舍，应该从表现文章主题的需要出发，分清主次，定好详略。要突出重点，详写细述那些能表现文章主题的重要情节，略写粗述那么非关键的次要情节。面面俱到反而使情节罗列化，使人不得要领。常见形式有：故事、日记、新闻报道、游记等。

Practice

Instructions：请你以假期旅行为题材写一篇记叙文，内容包含游览的时间、地点以及旅行过程中发生的难忘经历。

Unit Four
Diet

Guidance

1. This unit consists of Text A, Text B and Further Study. **Text A** tells us the importance of a healthy diet. **Text B** illustrates the phenomenon of food addiction. **Further Study** focuses on communication skills in terms of offering the help.

2. By learning this unit, students will be able to master the structure of the texts, new words, phrases and expressions. Students will improve their understanding of grammatical structures, reading comprehension and enlarge their vocabulary by doing the relevant exercises. Meanwhile, they will gain better understanding on *Diet*.

3. **Further Study** aims to improve students' skills for communication. By doing the exercises, students will know the differences in communication between Chinese and Westerners. They will perform well in everyday conversation and writing by doing this part.

> One cannot think well, love well, sleep well, if one has not dined well.
>
> — Virginia Woolf

▪▪ Text A   Healthy Diet

Anonymous

A healthy diet is one that helps maintain or improve general health. A healthy diet provides the body with essential nutrition: fluid, adequate essential amino acids from

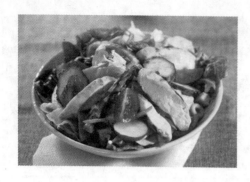

protein, essential fatty acids, vitamins, minerals, and adequate calories. The requirements for a healthy diet can be met from a variety of plant-based and animal-based foods. A healthy diet supports energy needs and provides for human nutrition without exposure to toxicity or excessive weight gain from consuming excessive amounts. Where lack of calories is not an issue, a properly balanced diet（in addition to exercise）is also thought to be important for lowering health risks, such as obesity, heart disease, type 2 diabetes[1], hypertension and cancer.

Various nutrition guides are published by medical and governmental institutions to educate the public on what they should be eating to promote health. Nutrition facts labels are also mandatory in some countries to allow consumers to choose between foods based on the components relevant to health.

For specific conditions

In addition to dietary recommendations for the general population, there are many specific diets that have primarily been developed to promote better health in specific population groups, such as people with high blood pressure, or people who are overweight or obese. However, some of them may have more or less evidence for beneficial effects in normal people as well.

Hypertension

A low sodium diet is beneficial for people with high blood pressure. The DASH diet （Dietary Approaches to Stop Hypertension）is a diet promoted by the National Heart, Lung, and Blood Institute（part of the NIH[2], a United States government organization）to control hypertension. A major feature of the plan is limiting intake of sodium, and it also generally encourages the consumption of nuts, whole grains, fish, poultry, fruits and vegetables while lowering the consumption of red meats, sweets, and sugar. It is also "rich in potassium, magnesium, and calcium, as well as protein". Evidence shows that[3] the Mediterranean diet[4] improves cardiovascular outcomes. WHO[5] recommends few standards such as an intake of less than 5 grams per person per day so as to prevent one from cardiovascular disease. Unsaturated fatty acids with polyunsaturated vegetable oils, on the other hand plays an essential role in reducing coronary heart disease risk as well as diabetes.

Weight control diets aim to maintain a controlled weight. In most cases dieting is used in combination with physical exercise to lose weight in those who are overweight or obese.

Diets to promote weight loss are divided into four categories: low-fat, low-carbohydrate, low-calorie, and very low calorie.

Reduced disease risk

There may be a relationship between lifestyle including food consumption and potentially lowering the risk of cancer or other chronic diseases. A diet high in fruits and vegetables appears to decrease the risk of cardiovascular disease and death but not cancer. A healthy diet may consist mostly of whole plant foods, with limited consumption of energy dense foods, red meat, alcoholic drinks and salt while reducing consumption of sugary drinks, and processed meat. A healthy diet may contain non-starchy vegetables and fruits[6], including those with red, green, yellow, white, purple or orange pigments. Tomato cooked with oil, allium vegetables like garlic, and cruciferous vegetables like cauliflower "probably" contain compounds which are under research for their possible anti-cancer activity. A healthy diet is low in energy density, lowering caloric content, thereby possibly inhibiting weight gain and lowering risk against chronic diseases.

New Words

amino /əˈmiːnəʊ/   *adj*. pertaining to or containing any of a group of organic compounds of nitrogen derived from ammonia 氨基的

fatty /ˈfætɪ/   *adj*. containing or consisting of fat 含脂肪的

mineral /ˈmɪnərəl/   *n*. a substance such as tin, salt, or sulphur that is formed naturally in rocks and in the earth 矿物质

calory /ˈkælərɪ/   *n*. (or calorie) a unit for measuring the amount of energy that food will produce 卡(路里)

toxicity /tɒkˈsɪsətɪ/   *n*. the quality of being poisonous; the extent to which sth. is poisonous 毒性;毒力

obesity /əʊˈbiːsətɪ/   *n*. a condition in which someone is too fat in a way that is dangerous for their health 肥胖;肥胖症

mandatory /ˈmændət(ə)rɪ/   *adj*. needing to be done, followed or complied with, usually because of an official requirement 强制的;法定的;义务的

relevant /ˈreləvənt/   *adj*. ① closely connected with the subject you are discussing or the situation you are thinking about 紧密相关的;切题的 ② having ideas that are valuable and useful to people in their lives and work 有价值的;有意义的

dietary /ˈdaɪət(ə)rɪ/   *adj*. related to the foods that someone eats 饮食的

recommendation /ˌrekəmenˈdeɪʃ(ə)n/   *n*. ① an official suggestion about the best thing to do 正式建议;提议 ② the act of telling sb. that sth. is good or useful or that sb. would be suitable for a particular job, etc. 推荐;介绍 ③ a formal letter or statement that sb. would be suitable for a particular job, etc. 推荐信;求职介绍信

overweight /ˌəʊvə(r)ˈweɪt/   *adj*. having more body weight than is considered healthy for the person's height, build or age 超重的

obese /əʊˈbiːs/   *adj*. very fat, in a way that is not healthy 过分肥胖的;臃肿的

sodium /ˈsəʊdɪəm/   *n*. a chemical element; a soft silver-white metal that is found naturally only in compounds, such as salt 钠

intake /ˈɪnteɪk/   *n*. the amount of food, drink, etc. that you take into your body (食物、饮料等的)摄取量,吸入量

poultry /ˈpəʊltrɪ/   *n*. ① chickens, ducks and geese, kept for their meat or eggs 家禽

② meat from chickens, ducks and geese 禽的肉

potassium /pə'tæsɪəm/   *n.* a chemical element; a soft silver-white metal that exists mainly in compounds which are used in industry and farming 钾

magnesium /mæg'niːzɪəm/   *n.* a chemical element; a light, silver-white metal that burns with a bright white flame 镁

calcium /'kælsɪəm/   *n.* a chemical element; a soft silver-white metal that is found in bones, teeth and chalk 钙

Mediterranean /ˌmedɪtə'reɪnɪən/   *adj.* connected with the Mediterranean Sea or the countries and regions that surround it; typical of this area 地中海的

cardiovascular /ˌkɑː(r)dɪəʊ'væskjʊlə(r)/   *adj.* connected with the heart and the blood vessels (= the tubes that carry blood around the body) 心血管的

unsaturated /ʌn'sætʃəˌreɪtɪd/   *adj.* not saturated; capable of dissolving more of a substance at a given temperature 不饱和的

polyunsaturated /ˌpɒlɪʌn'sætʃəˌreɪtɪd/   *adj.* belonging to a class of fats, especially plant oils, that are less likely to be converted into cholesterol in the body 多不饱和的

coronary /'kɒrən(ə)rɪ/   *adj.* connected with the heart, particularly the arteries that take blood to the heart 冠状动脉的

potentially /pə'tenʃəlɪ/   *adv.* possibly true in the future, but not true now 潜在地

chronic /'krɒnɪk/   *adj.* lasting for a long time; difficult to cure or get rid of 长期的；慢性的；难以治愈（或根除）的

alcoholic /ˌælkə'hɒlɪk/   *adj.* ① connected with or containing alcohol 酒精的；含酒精的 ② caused by drinking alcohol 饮酒引起的

sugary /'ʃʊgərɪ/   *adj.* ① containing sugar; tasting of sugar 含糖的；甜的 ② seeming too full of emotion in a way that is not sincere （态度等）甜腻腻的；甜言蜜语的

processed /'prəsest/   *adj.* subjected to a special process or treatment 加工过的，经加工的

pigment /'pɪgmənt/   *n.* a substance that gives something a particular colour 颜料；色素

allium /'ælɪəm/   *n.* large genus of perennial and biennial pungent bulbous plants: garlic; leek; onion; chive; sometimes placed in family Alliaceae as the type genus 葱属植物

cruciferous /k'ruːsɪfərəs/   *adj.* of or relating to or belonging to the plant family Cruciferae 十字花科的

cauliflower /'kɔːlɪflaʊə(r)/   *n.* a large round vegetable that has a hard white centre surrounded by green leaves 花椰菜；菜花

compound /kəm'paʊnd/   *n.* ① a thing consisting of two or more separate things combined together 复合物；混合物 ② a substance formed by a chemical reaction of two or more elements in fixed amounts relative to each other 化合物

anti-cancer /ˌæntiː'kænsə/   *adj.* used in the treatment of cancer 抗癌的

inhibit /ɪn'hɪbɪt/   *vt.* ① to prevent sth. from happening or make it happen more slowly or less frequently than normal 阻止；阻碍；抑制 ② to make sb. nervous or embarrassed so that they are unable to do sth. 使拘束；使尴尬

Phrases and Expressions

relevant to	与……有关的
more or less	或多或少
be beneficial for	有利于
aim to do sth.	打算做某事
in combination with	与……联合，与……结合

Text Notes

1. **Type 2 diabetes** is a lifelong（chronic）disease in which there is a high level of sugar（glucose）in the blood. Type 2 diabetes is the most common form of diabetes.
2. NIH（National Institutes of Health），即美国国立卫生研究院。
3. Evidence shows that...意为"证据表明……"，类似的表达有 Research/Study shows that...（研究表明……）和 Statistics shows that...（数据表明……）等。
4. **The Mediterranean diet** is a modern nutritional recommendation originally inspired by the traditional dietary patterns of Greece，Southern Italy，and Spain. The principal aspects of this diet include proportionally high consumption of olive oil，legumes，unrefined cereals，fruits，and vegetables，moderate to high consumption of fish，moderate consumption of dairy products（mostly as cheese and yogurt），moderate wine consumption，and low consumption of meat and meat products.
5. WHO，即 World Health Organization，世界卫生组织。
6. non-starchy vegetables and fruits 指的是"不含淀粉的蔬菜和水果"。

Text Comprehension

Please choose the best answers to the following questions according to the text.

1. The necessities of a healthy diet can be achieved from _____.
   A. adequate essential amino acids from protein
   B. a variety of plant-based and animal-based foods
   C. a properly balanced diet
   D. various nutrition guides
2. It is helpful for the people with hypertension to have a _____ diet.
   A. high sodium   B. low sodium
   C. high calcium   D. low calcium
3. It is shown by the evidence that the Mediterranean diet _____.
   A. is unhealthy
   B. can lead to cardiovascular disease
   C. is helpful for people with cardiovascular disease
   D. is tasty and healthy
4. Which of the following statements is NOT true?

A. Dieting is usually used together with exercise to lose weight.

B. A diet rich in fruits and vegetables usually decrease the risk of cardiovascular disease and cancer.

C. A healthy diet may contain mostly whole plant foods.

D. Unsaturated fatty acids with polyunsaturated vegetable oils are good for people's health.

5. From the passage, we know that a healthy diet _____.

A. is high in energy density

B. is high in caloric content

C. provides the body with essential nutrition

D. may cause excessive weight gain

Vocabulary and Structure

Please choose the best answer for each of the following sentences.

1. The child is spoiled by the _____ love from the grandparents.

  A. sufficient   B. moderate

  C. adequate   D. excessive

2. Oxygen is often stored as a liquid, although it is used _____ as a gas.

  A. primarily   B. seldom

  C. rarely   D. sometimes

3. We were in the same college, _____ was male-only at that time.

  A. that   B. which

  C. it   D. although

4. The commission is made up of five people, _____ two women.

  A. including   B. involving

  C. included   D. involved

5. All the windows _____ have been repaired.

  A. breaking   B. being broken

  C. broken   D. broke

Comprehensive Exercise

There are five incomplete sentences in the following passage. Read the passage and choose the word that best fits into the passage. Do remember each word can be used only once.

A. of	B. as	C. on	D. up	E. between

    Fears of high cholesterol were frequently voiced __1__ until the mid-1990s. However, more recent research has shown that the distinction __2__ high- and low-density lipoprotein ("good" and "bad" cholesterol, respectively) must be addressed when speaking __3__ the potential ill effects of cholesterol. Different types of dietary fat have different effects __4__ blood levels of cholesterol. For example, polyunsaturated fats tend to decrease both types of cholesterol; monounsaturated fats tend to lower LDL and raise HDL; saturated fats tend to either raise HDL, or raise both HDL and

LDL; and trans fat tend to raise LDL and lower HDL. Dietary cholesterol itself is only found in animal products such __5__ meat, eggs, and dairy, but studies have shown that even large amounts of dietary cholesterol only have negligible effects on blood cholesterol.

Translation

Please translate the following sentences into Chinese.

1. Everybody felt more or less thirsty.
2. All evidence relevant to this trial must be given to the police.
3. We are constantly being reminded to cut down our fat intake.
4. Obesity is a major risk factor in many diseases.
5. He speaks English and Spanish as well.

▪▪ Text B　Food Addiction

Anonymous

The idea that a person can be addicted to food has recently gotten more support from science.

Experiments in animals and humans show that[1], for some people, the same reward and pleasure centers of the brain that are triggered by addictive drugs like cocaine and heroin are also activated by food, especially highly palatable foods. Highly palatable foods are foods rich in: sugar, fat and salt.

Like addictive drugs, highly palatable foods trigger feel-good[2] brain chemicals such as dopamine. Once people experience pleasure associated with increased dopamine transmission in the brain's reward pathway from eating certain foods, they quickly feel the need to eat again.

The reward signals from highly palatable foods may override other signals of fullness and satisfaction. As a result, people keep eating, even when they're not hungry.

People who show signs of food addiction may also develop a tolerance to food. They eat more and more, only to find that food satisfies them less and less.

Scientists believe that food addiction may play an important role in obesity. But normal-weight people[3] may also struggle with food addiction. Their bodies may simply be genetically programmed to better handle the extra calories they take in. Or they may increase their physical activity to compensate for overeating.

People who are addicted to food will continue to eat despite negative consequences, such as weight gain or damaged relationships. And like people who are addicted to drugs or gambling, people who are addicted to food will have trouble stopping their behavior, even if they want to or have tried many times to cut back.

Signs of Food Addiction

Researchers at Yale University's Rudd Center for Food Science & Policy have developed a questionnaire to identify people with food addictions.

Here's a sample of questions that can help determine if you have a food addiction. Do these actions apply to you? Do you:

End up eating more than planned when you start eating certain foods

Keep eating certain foods even if you're no longer hungry

Eat to the point of feeling ill

Worry about not eating certain types of foods or worry about cutting down on certain types of foods

When certain foods aren't available, go out of your way[4] to obtain them

The questionnaire also asks about the impact of your relationship with food on your personal life. Do these situations apply to you?

You eat certain foods so often or in such large amounts that you start eating food instead of working, spending time with the family, or doing recreational activities.

You avoid professional or social situations where certain foods are available because of fear of overeating.

You have problems functioning effectively at your job or school because of food and eating.

The questionnaire asks about withdrawal symptoms[5]. For example, when you cut down on certain foods (excluding caffeinated beverages), do you have symptoms such as: anxiety and agitation.

The questionnaire also tries to gauge the impact of food decisions on your emotions. Do these situations apply to you?

Eating food causes problems such as depression, anxiety, self-loathing, or guilt.

You need to eat more and more food to reduce negative emotions or increase pleasure.

Eating the same amount of food doesn't reduce negative emotions or increase pleasure the way it used to.

New Words

addiction /əˈdɪkʃ(ə)n/   *n.* the condition of being addicted to sth. 瘾;入迷;嗜好

addictive /əˈdɪktɪv/   *adj.* making or likely to make somebody an addict 使人上瘾的

cocaine /kəʊˈkeɪn/   *n.* a powerful drug that some people take illegally for pleasure and can become addicted to, and doctors sometimes use it as an anaesthetic 可卡因

heroin /ˈhɛrəʊɪn/   *n.* a powerful illegal drug made from morphine, that some people take for pleasure and can become addicted to 海洛因

activate /ˈæktɪveɪt/   *vt.* to make sth. such as a device or chemical process start working 使活动;激活;使活化

palatable /ˈpælətəb(ə)l/   *adj.* ① having a pleasant or acceptable taste 可口的;味美的 ② pleasant or acceptable to sb. 宜人的;可意的;可接受的

dopamine /ˈdəʊpəmiːn/   *n.* a chemical produced by nerve cells which has an effect on other cells 多巴胺(神经细胞产生的一种作用于其他细胞的化学物质)

pathway /ˈpɑːθˌweɪ/   *n*. a path or a route 道路；路径

override /ˌəʊvəˈraɪd/   *vt*. ① to use your authority to reject sb.'s decision, order, etc. （以权力）否决；推翻；不理会   ② to be more important than sth. 比……更重要；凌驾   ③ to stop a process that happens automatically and control it yourself 超驰控制；超控（使自动控制暂时失效，改用手工控制）

     n. An override is an attempt to cancel someone's decisions by using your authority over them or by gaining more votes than them in an election or contest （对决定等的）撤销；推翻；否决

genetically /dʒəˈnetɪklɪ/   *adv*. in a way that is connected with genetics 遗传学上

overeating /ˌəʊvərˈiːtɪŋ/   *n*. eating to excess 暴食；吃得过量

gambling /ˈɡæmblɪŋ/   *n*. the act of playing for stakes in the hope of winning (including the payment of a price for a chance to win a prize) 赌博；赌钱

questionnaire /ˌkwestʃəˈneə(r)/   *n*. a written list of questions that are answered by a number of people so that information can be collected from the answers 调查表；问卷

recreational /ˌrekrɪˈeɪʃ(ə)n(ə)l/   *adj*. connected with activities that people do for enjoyment when they are not working 娱乐的；消遣的

withdrawal /wɪðˈdrɔːəl/   *n*. ① the act or process of removing it, or ending it 收回；撤回；停止   ② an amount of money that you take from your bank 取款；提款

symptom /ˈsɪmptəm/   *n*. ① a change in your body or mind that shows that you are not healthy 症状   ② a sign that sth. exists, especially sth. bad 征候；征兆

caffeinated /ˈkæfɪneɪtɪd/   *adj*. containing caffeine 含有咖啡因的

beverage /ˈbev(ə)rɪdʒ/   *n*. any type of drink except water （除水以外的）饮料

agitation /ˌædʒɪˈteɪʃ(ə)n/   *n*. ① worry and anxiety that you show by behaving in a nervous way 焦虑不安；忧虑；烦乱   ② public protest in order to achieve political change 骚动；煽动；鼓动   ③ the act of stirring or shaking a liquid （液体的）搅动；摇动

gauge /ɡeɪdʒ/   *n*. ① an instrument for measuring the amount or level of sth. 测量仪器（或仪表）；计量器   ② a measurement of the width or thickness of sth. 宽度；厚度   ③ a fact or an event that can be used to estimate or judge sth. （用于估计或判断的）事实；依据；尺度；标准

self-loathing /ˈselfˈləʊðɪŋ/   *n*. the feeling of hating oneself 自我讨厌

Phrases and Expressions

be addicted to   沉迷于

struggle with   与……斗争

take in   吸收；领会

compensate for	赔偿；补偿损失
have trouble doing sth.	做某事有困难
cut back	削减
apply to	适用于；运用
end up doing	以（做）……而告终
cut down on	减少；节省

Text Notes

1. Experiments...show that，意思是"实验表明……"。

2. feel-good，即 making you feel happy and pleased about life，意为"使人愉悦的"，动词短语 feel good 表示"感觉良好"。

3. normal-weight people 指"体重正常的人"。

4. go out of one's way 指"特意不怕麻烦做某事，不厌其烦"。例如：They went out of their way to help us. 他们特地来帮助我们。

5. withdrawal symptoms 指的是"脱隐症状或戒断症状（戒除某习惯时所引起的痛苦和不适）"。例如：If these drugs are stopped abruptly, then some withdrawal symptoms may occur. 如果突然停服这些药，则可能出现一些戒断症状。

Text Comprehension

Please read the following statements and mark T/F according to the text.

1. Highly palatable foods are usually sugary, fatty and salty.
   A. T   B. F

2. Highly palatable foods make people feel good and may quickly feel the need to eat again.
   A. T   B. F

3. Food addiction has nothing to do with obesity.
   A. T   B. F

4. Normal-weight people are less likely to suffer from food addiction.
   A. T   B. F

5. If someone has problems functioning effectively at his or her job or school due to food and eating, he or she may have food addiction.
   A. T   B. F

Vocabulary and Structure

Please complete the following sentences with the proper forms of the words given.

1. Cigarettes are highly _____ . (addict)

2. Please note that the goods you ordered can be promised for immediate shipment upon receipt of payment, _____ Sundays and holidays. (exclude)

3. She had no _____ for jokes of any kind. (tolerant)

4. She felt a glow of _____ at her son's achievements. (satisfy)

5. The public should be educated to use resources more _____ . (effective)

Translation

Please translate the following passage into Chinese.

Compulsive overeating, also sometimes called food addiction, is characterized by an obsessive/compulsive relationship to food. Left untreated, compulsive overeating can lead to serious medical conditions including high cholesterol, diabetes, heart disease, hypertension, sleep apnea, and major depression. Additional long-term side effects of the condition also include kidney disease, arthritis, bone deterioration and stroke.

■■ Further Study

（Offering the Help）

提供帮助(Offering the Help)：提供帮助是人们在日常生活中经常会遇到的一种场景,它往往具有特定的语言表达形式。询问对方是否需要帮助时通常用疑问句,对方可以接受帮助或委婉拒绝。

Key Sentences

◆ Offering the help
○ Can I help you?
○ May I help you?
○ What can I do for you?
○ Can I help you with ...?
○ Can I help you to ...?
○ Is there anything I can do for you?
○ Would you like some help with ...?
◆ Responses to the offering of help
○ That's very kind of you.
○ It's very kind of you.
○ I appreciate it very much.
○ Thank you very much for...
○ No, thanks. I can manage it myself.
○ That's Ok, I can handle it myself.

Practice

1. — Can I help you?

— _____ .

A. That's right   B. No, thanks

C. Here you are   D. Yes, I can

2. — _____

— Yes，where is ladies' room please?

A．I can help you. B．Let me help you.

C．May I help you? D．What can I do for you?

3. — May I help you?

— _____．

A．Yes，you can B．Sorry

C．Yes，please D．No，you can't

4. — May I help you?

— _____．I want to visit the Summer Palace and the Tsinghua University.

A．Yes B．Of course

C．No D．Never mind

5. — Can I help you? What would you like?

— I don't know.

— Would you like something to eat? How about some cakes?

— _____．I think I'd like some bread.

A．Yes，please B．That's it

C．No，thanks D．It doesn't matter

Grammar

> 状语从句(Adverbial Clause)：状语从句指句子用作状语时，起副词作用的句子。它可以修饰谓语、非谓语动词、定语、状语或整个句子。根据其作用可分为时间、地点、原因、条件、目的、结果、让步、方式和比较等从句。状语从句一般由连词(从属连词)引导，也可以由词组引导。从句位于句首或句中时通常用逗号与主句隔开，位于句尾时可以不用逗号隔开。

一、时间状语从句

常用引导词：when(在……时)，as(当……时)，while(在……期间)，as soon as(一……就……)，before(在……之前)，after(在……之后)，since(自从……以来)，not...until(直到……才)

特殊引导词：the minute，the moment，the second，every time，the day，the instant(瞬间，顷刻)，immediately，directly(不久，立即)，no sooner ... than(一……就……)，hardly ... when(刚一……就……)，scarcely ... when(几乎没有……的时候)

例如：While John was watching TV，his wife was cooking.

当约翰看电视时，他的妻子正在做饭。

No sooner had I arrived home than it began to rain.

我一到家就开始下雨了。

二、地点状语从句

常用引导词：where

特殊引导词：wherever，anywhere，everywhere

例如：Generally，air will be heavily polluted where there are factories.

一般来说,有工厂的地方空气污染就严重。

Wherever you go, you should work hard.

无论你去哪里,你都应该努力工作。

三、原因状语从句

常用引导词:because, since, as, for

特殊引导词:seeing that, now that, in that, considering that, given that

例如:Now that everybody has come, let's begin our conference.

既然每个人都到了,让我们开始会议吧。

四、目的状语从句

常用引导词:so that, in order that

特殊引导词:lest, in case, for fear that, in the hope that, for the purpose that, to the end that

例如:The teacher raised his voice on purpose that the students in the back could hear more clearly.

为了让后面的学生听得更清楚,老师有意地提高了他的声音。

五、结果状语从句

常用引导词:so ... that, such ... that

特殊引导词:such that, to the degree that, to the extent that, to such a degree that

例如:It's such a good chance that we must not miss it.

这是一个好机会,千万不能错过它。

六、条件状语从句

常用引导词:if, unless, whether (whether...or not)

特殊引导词:as/so long as, only if, providing/provided that, supposing that, in case that, on condition that

例如:We'll start our project if the president agrees.

如果总统同意,我们将开始我们的项目。

You will certainly succeed so long as you keep on trying.

只要你继续努力,你一定会成功的。

Provided that there is no opposition, we shall hold the meeting here.

如果没有人反对,我们就在这里开会。

七、让步状语从句

常用引导词:though, although, even if, even though

特殊引导词:as(用在让步状语从句中必须要倒装),while（一般用在句首）,no matter ... , in spite of the fact that, whatever, whoever, wherever, whenever, however, whichever

例如:No matter how hard he tried, she could not change her mind.

不论他如何努力,她都不会改变她的主意。

He won't listen whatever you may say.

无论你说什么他都不会听。

八、比较状语从句

常用引导词:as(同级比较),than(不同程度的比较)

特殊引导词:the more ... the more ...;just as ...,so...;A is to B what/as X is to Y;no ... more than; not so much A as B

例如:The house is three times as big as ours.

这房子是我们的三倍大。

The more you exercise, the healthier you will be.

你运动得越多,你就越健康。

九、方式状语从句

常用引导词:as, as if, how

特殊引导词:the way

例如:When in Rome, do as the Romans do.

入国问禁,入乡随俗。

Sometimes we teach our children the way our parents have taught us.

有时,我们用父母教导我们的方式教导孩子。

Practice

1. _____ there is no rain, farming is difficult or impossible.
   A. As   B. Though
   C. Where   D. When

2. He got up _____ early _____ he caught the first bus.
   A. so; as to   B. so; that
   C. as; as   D. such; that

3. _____ I respect him, I can't agree to his proposal.
   A. As   B. Provided
   C. Because   D. Much as

4. She behaved _____ she were the boss.
   A. as   B. as if
   C. even if   D. even though

5. Food is to men _____ oil is to machine.
   A. what   B. that
   C. which   D. in which

Writing

议论文是作者对某个问题或某件事进行分析、评论,表明自己的观点、立场、态度、看法和主张的一种文体。议论文有三要素,即论点、论据和论证。论点的基本要求是:观点正确,认真概括,有实际意义;论据的基本要求是:真实可靠,充分典型;论证的基本要求是:推理必须符合逻辑。

英语议论文的结构一般较为固定,通常包括以下三部分:

1. 在导语部分提出需要议论的议题;

2. 在正文部分对所提出的问题进行议论;

3. 在结论部分对以上的讨论进行总结和归纳。

在具体写作中要注意下列几点:

1. 议题的提出要开门见山,不要拖泥带水;

2. 议论时可以采用不同的方法。如:可以摆出正反两方面观点,进行对比;也可引经据典论证作者自己观点的正确性,从而使读者接受自己的观点;亦可提出一种错误的观点然后论证其错误,最终提出正确的观点。正文部分是写作的重点,论证方法可用归纳法、推理法、比较法等;

3. 在结论部分必须表明作者的观点,对讨论的问题做出总结;

4. 注意连接词和过渡词等词语的使用,以增强文章的条理性和逻辑性。常用的过渡词和连接词包括:first, second, third, finally, in addition, furthermore, besides, what was worse, more importantly, in contrast, because, since, now that, therefore, consequently, in that case, as a result/consequence, in conclusion, to sum up 等等。

Practice

Instructions: *There are five incomplete sentences in the following passage. Read the passage and choose the word that best fits into the passage. Do remember each word can be used only once.*

> A. As a result B. Furthermore C. In conclusion D. Second E. First of all

Shall We Send Children to Study Abroad?

With more and more people becoming rich in recent years, it is a new tendency for them to send their children to study abroad.

But I don't think it is a good idea. _____, children are too young to look after themselves. _____, the language barrier is a serious problem. Many children are not proficient in the foreign language before going abroad. _____, they have difficulty in understanding what the native speakers are talking about. Third, they may get into trouble when dealing with various situations for lack of knowledge of the customs in the strange land. _____, the cost of living is much higher than that in our country, which might cause a heavy burden to the family.

_____, there are more disadvantages in sending children to study abroad. So, we'd better not do it.

Unit Five
Stress

- Healthy Lifestyle Habits for Stress Relief
- Back-to-School Stress Relief Techniques

Guidance

1. This unit consists of Text A, Text B and Further Study. **Text A** gives us suggestions on how to relieve stress by adopting healthy lifestyle habits. **Text B** is about how to deal with school-year stressors so as to help achieve academic success. **Further Study** focuses on communication skills in terms of making requests.

2. By learning this unit, students will be able to master the structure of the texts, new words, phrases and expressions. Students will improve their understanding of grammatical structures, reading comprehension and enlarge their vocabulary by doing the relevant exercises. Meanwhile, they will gain better understanding on relieving *Stress*.

3. **Further Study** aims to improve students' skills for communication. By doing the exercises, students will know the differences in communication between Chinese and Westerners. They will perform well in everyday conversation and writing by doing this part.

Stress is the trash of modern life. We all generate it, but if you don't dispose of it properly, it will pile up and overtake your life.

— Terri Guillemets

■■ Text A   Healthy Lifestyle Habits for Stress Relief

Elizabeth Scott, M. S[1]

We all experience stress. And, just as[2] stress comes from many areas of life, effective stress management comes from combating stress on many different fronts.

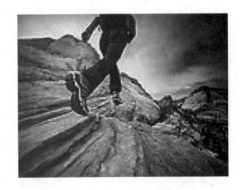

Part of a comprehensive stress relief plan involves finding ways to calm down quickly so you can more effectively manage stress as it comes, while[3] avoiding the negative effects of chronic stress. Another important way to relieve stress is to maintain healthy lifestyle habits. Maintaining a balanced, healthy lifestyle is important.

While[3] maintaining healthy habits is a bit more challenging than trying a stress relief method only once, the benefits you receive from maintaining a healthy lifestyle are more than worth the effort it takes to maintain it. The increases in health and wellness that you experience, and the reduction in stress, will make you wish you'd made these changes sooner, and can be wonderful sources of continued motivation.

Many people feel intimidated by making healthy lifestyle changes for a few reasons: There are so many changes that can benefit health and wellness that it's difficult to know where to[4] start. People often try to make too many changes at once, then find it too difficult (or let perfectionism sabotage their efforts), and give up the effort. Let's face it: change is difficult, especially when you're stressed. Sometimes lifestyle stress takes over and diminishes momentum.

Given[5] that living a healthy lifestyle can help with stress relief, and that making healthy lifestyle changes can be challenging, the following resources can help you with both choosing new goals for healthy living, and making these new goals a reality, and adopting new healthy habits into your lifestyle.

The following are some changes you can make to lead a healthier, less stressed lifestyle.

Healthy Eating. One of the most popular changes people like to make to live a healthy lifestyle is to eat differently. Because of the negative health consequences of obesity, the influence fitness has on our self-esteem, and the effects of nutrition on our stress levels and longevity, switching to a healthier diet brings some of the greatest benefits for wellness. Read about stress and weight gain, the interaction between stress and nutrition or the role of stress in emotional eating.

Regular Exercise. Getting regular exercise is another wonderful way to keep your weight in check, manage overall stress levels, and stay connected with others. Exercise can also help keep many health conditions at bay, and is well worth the effort. (The trick is to start gradually and work your way up.) Learn more about exercise for stress relief, and find exercise tips for busy people.

Quality Sleep. People often underestimate the importance of getting enough sleep, and getting the right type. However, lack of adequate sleep has many negative consequences — they're subtle, but significant. Getting enough sleep isn't one of the most popular changes that people resolve to make, but it should be. Because stress can rob you of sleep, and because many of the techniques that promote sleep can also reduce stress (and vice versa[6]), it's a very good idea to learn more about how stress affects sleep and how to get quality sleep when stressed.

New Words

comprehensive /ˌkɒmprɪˈhensɪv/	*adj*. including many, most, or all things 全面的；综合的；包罗万象的；详尽的
relief /rɪˈliːf/	*n*. a feeling of happiness that something unpleasant has not happened or has ended（不快过后的）宽慰，宽心，轻松，解脱
negative /ˈnegətɪv/	*adj*. lacking in definite, constructive or helpful qualities or characteristics 消极的；无助益的
wellness /ˈwelnəs/	*n*. the state of being healthy 健康
reduction /rɪˈdʌkʃən/	*n*. when you make or when something becomes smaller in size, amount, degree, importance 减少；减小；降低；缩小
motivation /ˌməʊtɪˈveɪʃən/	*n*. enthusiasm for doing something 积极性；干劲
intimidate /ɪnˈtɪmɪdeɪt/	*vt*. to frighten or threaten someone, usually in order to persuade them to do something that you want them to do 恫吓，恐吓
perfectionism /pəˈfekʃənɪzəm/	*n*. the wish for everything to be correct 至善论，完美主义
sabotage /ˈsæbətɑːʒ/	*vt*. to damage or destroy equipment, weapons or buildings in order to prevent the success of an enemy or competitor（为阻止敌人或对手成功而）毁坏，破坏（设备、武器或建筑物）
diminish /dɪˈmɪnɪʃ/	*vt*. to reduce or be reduced in size or importance 减少，减小，降低
momentum /məˈmentəm/	*n*. the force that keeps an object moving or keeps an event developing after it has started 动量，冲量；冲力；推动力；势头
self-esteem /ˈselfɪˈstiːm/	*n*. belief and confidence in your own ability and value 自尊
nutrition /njuːˈtrɪʃən/	*n*. the substances that you take into your body as food and the way that they influence your health 营养物质；营养，滋养
underestimate /ˌʌndəˈestɪmeɪt/	*vt*. to fail to guess or understand the real cost, size, difficulty, etc. of something 低估；（对……）估计不足
subtle /ˈsʌtl/	*adj*. not loud, bright, noticeable or obvious in any way 隐约的；暗淡的；不易察觉的，不明显的；微妙的
promote /prəˈməʊt/	*vt*. to encourage the popularity, sale, development or existence of something 促进；促销，推销，推广

Phrases and Expressions

calm down	（使）平静；（使）冷静；（使）镇静
take over	接任；接管，接手
keep ... in check	抑制；约束；制止
keep ... at bay	阻止，遏制（令人不快的事物）

Text Notes

1. **Elizabeth Scott，M. S** is a stress management expert，wellness coach，author，health educator，and award-winning blogger with training in counseling，family therapy，and health psychology.

2. **just as** 为"正如……"之意。例如：One day she will walk out，just as her own mother did. 总有一天她会离家出走，就像她母亲那样。又如：He died of cancer just as his father did. 他死于癌症，就像他父亲那样。

3. **while** 此处为连词，表示"在……期间""与……同时""虽然""而……"。例如：Jim Coulters will mind the store while I'm away. 我不在的时候吉姆·库尔特斯会照看店铺的。又如：While I fully understand your point of view，I do also have some sympathy with Michael's. 尽管我完全能理解你的观点，但我在一定程度上也赞同迈克尔的观点。又如：Tom is very extrovert and confident while Katy's shy and quiet. 汤姆性格外向，非常自信，而凯蒂却羞涩文静。

4. **where to start** 表示"从哪里开始"。where to(do)为疑问代词或疑问副词＋to＋动词原形的结构。例如：She didn't know what to say. 她不知道说什么。又如：Jim asked his father how to make a model plane. 吉姆问父亲如何做一架模型飞机。

5. **given** 表示"考虑到""鉴于"。例如：Given his age，he's a remarkably fast runner. 考虑到他的年龄，他可称得上是个很出众的赛跑运动员了。又如：Given (the fact) that he's had six months to do this，he hasn't made much progress. 鉴于他有六个月做这件事，他取得的进展并不大。

6. **and vice versa** 表示"反过来也一样""反之亦然"。例如：He doesn't trust her，and vice versa (＝ she also doesn't trust him). 他不信任她，她也一样不信任他。

Text Comprehension

Please choose the best answers to the following questions according to the text.

1. Maintaining healthy habits is a bit more challenging，_____ .
   A. so you should only try a stress relief method once
   B. but you should maintain healthy habits.
   C. so you should not maintain healthy habits.
   D. but you shouldn't try a stress relief method.

2. What does the word "intimidated" mean in Para. 4?
   A. Frightened.　　　B. Resisted.　　　C. Reluctant.　　　D. Persisted.

3. Which of the following is TRUE according to the passage?
   A. Sometimes lifestyle stress takes over and increases momentum.
   B. Living a healthy lifestyle can help with stress relief.
   C. The most popular change people like to make to live a healthy lifestyle is to eat differently.
   D. People overestimate the importance of getting enough sleep.

4. It's a very good idea to learn more about how stress affects sleep and how to get quality sleep when stressed, because _____ .

    A. stress can rob you of sleep

    B. many of the techniques that promote sleep can also reduce stress (and vice versa)

    C. lack of adequate sleep has many negative consequences

    D. all of the above

5. What is the author's purpose of writing this passage?

    A. To introduce effective ways to stay healthy.

    B. To stress the importance of sleep.

    C. To advise people to maintain healthy lifestyle habits to combat stress.

    D. To make an advertisement for some stress relief products.

Vocabulary and Structure

Please choose the best answer for each of the following sentences.

1. If you have a _____ diet, you are getting all the vitamins you need.

    A. balanced   B. bankrupt

    C. biased   D. boring

2. People often try to make too many changes _____ , then find it too difficult.

    A. at least   B. at once

    C. at most   D. at all

3. You'll never guess the answer. Do you _____ ?

    A. give up   B. get off

    C. give away   D. get down

4. _____ I accept that he's not perfect in many respects, I do actually quite like the man.

    A. why   B. how

    C. who   D. while

5. Obsessive _____ can be very irritating.

    A. perfectionism   B. awareness

    C. person   D. critic

Comprehensive Exercise

There are five incomplete sentences in the following passage. Read the passage and choose the word that best fits into the passage. Do remember each word can be used only once.

> A. from   B. to   C. as   D. or   E. on

    Just __1__ there are different types of stress, there are different types of people, and some are more reactive __2__ stress than others. Because the body's stress response is triggered by perceived threat (rather than actual threat), the body's ability to return to homeostasis, __3__ its normal state, also varies __4__ person to person, with some people calming down immediately and others remaining overstimulated for hours after a stress trigger. Certain personality types also tend to bring

___5___ more stress, and respond to stressful situations less effectively, such as perfectionists or those who are "Type A".

Translation

Please translate the following sentences into Chinese.

1. He took over from the previous headmaster in February.
2. Exercise can help keep fat at bay.
3. We must find ways of keeping our expenditure in check.
4. She sat down and took a few deep breaths to calm herself down.
5. She's been feeling very stressed since she started her new job.

■■ Text B Back-to-School Stress Relief Techniques

Elizabeth Scott, M. S

While many families experience stress during the summer, there's no denying that the school year brings a unique set of stressors that can take a physical and psychological toll on all family members. When school is in session, it helps immensely to have a plan! The following are some of the proven ways to relieve school-year stress and maximize your success, with resources from some of About. com's[1] best health experts.

Maintain a Healthy Diet — Even When Things Get Busy

It's no secret that poor nutrition can exacerbate stress, but studies also show that well-fed kids are more successful in school. Be sure to feed yourself and your family a healthy breakfast (even when your mornings are busy) and a healthy dinner (family dinners can be stress relievers in themselves), and be sure you're packing healthy lunches as well[2]. If you're a college student, learn how to avoid the "freshman 15" and develop healthy eating routines while you're at school. Your body will thank you for it, and you'll all feel less stressed as well.

Prioritize Sleep and Everything Will Seem Easier

Lack of sleep can make everything feel more stressful, and can affect your performance in everything from test-taking to driving a car. Getting enough sleep can be more challenging during the school year than during summer if it means you don't have to rush the family out of the house as early in the morning, or stay up late helping with homework. For college students, summer is usually one long break, but the school year can bring late nights and even all-nighters. Rest easier by prioritizing sleep, developing stress-relief strategies that help you to get better-quality sleep, and trouble-shoot those sleep saboteurs. Be sure to do the same for your kids, and the whole family should be happier and more efficient

Maintain Healthy Habits and Get Enough Exercise

Taking care of your body through exercise and other healthy habits can keep you and your family in better shape, which means higher energy levels, lower stress, and, most likely, a stronger bond. Play with your kids, make time to be active as a family, and be sure to incorporate healthy habits into your daily life.

Keep That Stress Managed!

Stress can deplete your energy, affect your memory, and generally make it more difficult to excel in school or manage the responsibilities that come with maintaining your status as a student or parent of students. Many stress relief activities can also enhance your health, and once[3] you get into the habit, these ideas can be an important and enjoyable part of your life. As a bonus[4], teaching your kids stress management techniques in their childhood can help them to stay healthier and happier as adults who know how to cope with stress.

Get Organized, and Stay Organized

It's much more stressful to scramble through your morning without a plan, or make up your nighttime routine on the fly[5]. Searching for lost items can eat up time, and living in clutter creates stress. It really pays to be organized.

Be Proactive If You Are a College Student

I should say "stay proactive", as you've already taken the initiative of reading this article, and are likely considering which changes you might want to put into action. Take things a step further by creating a specific plan for stress management, and following through on that plan.

New Words

toll /təʊl/	*n*. suffering, deaths or damage 伤亡;损失;破坏
session /ˈseʃən/	*n*. at a college, any of the periods of time that a teaching year or day is divided into, or the teaching year itself 学年;学期;上课时间
immensely /ɪˈmenslɪ/	*adv*. extremely 非常,极其
maximize /ˈmæksɪmaɪz/	*vt*. to make something as great in amount, size or importance as possible 使最大化;使最重要
exacerbate /ɪgˈzæsəbeɪt/	*vt*. to make something which is already bad worse 使恶化;使加重;使加剧
routine /ruːˈtiːn/	*n*. a usual or fixed way of doing things 惯例,常规;例行公事
prioritize /praɪˈɒrɪtaɪz/	*vt*. to decide which of a group of things are the most important so that you can deal with them first 确定(事项的)优先次序
all-nighter /ɔːlˈnaɪtə/	*n*. a time when you spend all night studying, esp. for an examination (尤指考试前的)通宵学习
strategy /ˈstrætədʒɪ/	*n*. a detailed plan or skill for achieving success 战略;策略;计谋;行动计划;策划,部署
troubleshooting /ˈtrʌblʃuːtɪŋ/	*n*. discovering why something does not work effectively and making suggestions about how to improve it 处理难题;调解;检修
saboteur /ˌsæbəˈtɜːr/	*n*. a person who sabotages something 破坏者,毁坏者
bond /bɒnd/	*n*. a close connection joining two or more people (亲近的)联系,

关系

deplete /dɪˈpliːt/	*vt*. to reduce something in size or amount，esp. supplies of energy, money, etc. 消耗；耗费；减少
status /ˈsteɪtəs/	*n*. an accepted or official position，esp. in a social group（尤指在社会中的）地位，身份
bonus /ˈbəʊnəs/	*n*. ① a pleasant extra thing 另外的优点；额外的好处 ② an extra amount of money that is given to you as a present or reward as well as the money you were expecting 奖金；红利
scramble /ˈskræmbl/	*vi*. ① to move or climb quickly but with difficulty（匆匆、急速而艰难地）移动；爬；攀登 ② to compete with other people for something there is very little of 争抢
clutter /ˈklʌtə/	*n*.（a lot of objects in）a state of being untidy 杂乱，凌乱；杂乱的东西
proactive /prəʊˈæktɪv/	*adj*. taking action by causing change and not only reacting to change when it happens 主动的，积极的
initiative /ɪˈnɪʃətɪv/	*adv*. a new action or movement，often intended to solve a problem 倡议；新措施
specific /spəˈsɪfɪk/	*adj*. relating to one thing and not others；particular 特定的；特有的

Phrases and Expressions

in session	上课；开会
freshman 15	大一 15 磅，即新生在第一年中会增加 15 磅或者更多的体重
keep ... in better shape	保持更好的身材
live in clutter	生活在混乱中
follow through	坚持到底；完成球棒击球后的弧形动作

Text Notes

1. About. Com 创建于 1997 年，是美国纽约时报集团旗下的一个进行分类信息推荐的生活服务类网站。

2. as well 表示"除……之外还""也""和"。例如：Invite Emlyn and Simon as well. 邀请埃姆琳还有西蒙。又如：I want to visit Andrew as well as Martin. 我想去拜访安德鲁，还有马丁。

3. once 表示"一……就""一旦……就"。例如：Once I've found somewhere to live I'll send you my address. 我一找到住的地方就把地址告诉你。又如：Remember that you won't be able to cancel the contract once you've signed. 记住一旦你签了字就不能取消合同了。

4. bonus 表示"另外的优点""额外的好处"。例如：I love the job, and it's an added bonus that it's so close to home. 我喜欢这份工作，它还有个优点是离家很近。

5. on the fly 表示"匆忙地""在百忙中"。例如：It was all pretty much done on the fly. 那几乎都是匆忙之中完成的。又如：We had so little time to catch the train that we had to eat our lunch on the fly. 离上火车的时间不多了，所以我们不得不匆忙地吃午饭。

Text Comprehension

Please read the following statements and mark T/F according to the text.

1. There's no denying that the school year brings a unique set of stressors that can take a physical and psychological toll on all family members

   A. T   B. F

2. It's no secret that poor nutrition can exacerbate stress, but studies also show that ill-fed kids are more successful in school.

   A. T   B. F

3. If you're a college student, you cannot learn to avoid the "freshman 15" or develop healthy eating routines while you're at school.

   A. T   B. F

4. Lack of sleep can make everything feel more stressful, but cannot affect your performance in everything from test-taking to driving a car.

   A. T   B. F

5. Rest easier by prioritizing sleep, developing stress-relief strategies that help you to get better-quality sleep.

   A. T   B. F

Vocabulary and Structure

Please complete the following sentences with the proper forms of the words given.

1. You must learn to _____ your work. (prior)
2. Some athletes take drugs to improve their _____. (perform)
3. Exercise has become part of my _____ routine. (day)
4. Rebecca always _____ in languages at school. (excellence)
5. The letters have been place in _____ piles. (organize)
6. The peace _____ was welcomed by both sides. (initiate)
7. This problem calls for prompt _____ from the government. (act)
8. The virus attacks _____ cells in the brain. (specify)

Translation

Please translate the following passage into Chinese.

Because exercise is such an effective activity for stress management, anything that can help you to become more active can also help you to feel less stressed. What's great about fitness trackers is that the mere act of tracking your fitness can help you to increase your activity; seeing your steps taken or minutes of activity or miles walked for the day can inspire you to go just a little bit further — and then a little further.

▋▋ Further Study

（Making Requests）

Communication Skills

请求（Making Requests）：提出请求的方式按照客气和委婉程度可分为直接请求和间接请求。一般说来，提出请求的方式越间接（委婉），就显得越礼貌。回答请求（尤其是否定回答）也要注意直接性和间接性。一般说来间接委婉的拒绝请求要比直接拒绝显得客气有礼貌。

Key Sentences

◆ Making requests

○ Could I borrow your umbrella?

○ Would you do me a favor?

○ May I have a word with you?

○ Would you mind my smoking here?

○ Would you be so kind as to help us with it?

○ May I ask a favor of you?

○ Could you possibly explain that again?

○ Do you think I could take this one?

○ I wonder if you could help me with it?

○ Is it all right if I open the window?

○ Pass the dictionary, will you?

○ Please pass me the salt.

○ No smoking, please.

◆ Replies to requests

○ Sure.

○ Certainly.

○ All right.

○ OK.

○ By all means.

○ With pleasure.

○ I'll be glad to.

○ Yes, please do.

○ Yes. Go ahead.

○ No, I'm afraid you can't.

○ No, I'm afraid I can't.

○ I'm sorry, but you can't.

○ I'm sorry, but I'm using it right now.

○ Well, I'd like to, but....

Practice

1. — Could you do me a favor?
   — _____

   A. Never mind.　　　　　　　　B. With pleasure.
   C. Can't complain.　　　　　　D. Not at all.

2. — Could you stay a little longer?
   — _____

   A. No, I'm afraid I can't.　　　B. Yes, thank you.
   C. No, thank you.　　　　　　D. You are welcome.

3. — Would you please come over?
   — _____

   A. Sure.　　　　　　　　　　B. Right.
   C. Yes, please do.　　　　　　D. Well.

4. — I wonder if I could use your bike?
   — _____

   A. No.　　　　　　　　　　　B. None.
   C. Thanks.　　　　　　　　　D. I'm sorry, but I'm using it right now.

5. — Pass the dictionary, will you?
   — _____

   A. By all means.　　　　　　　B. Pleasure.
   C. None.　　　　　　　　　　D. Thanks.

Grammar

英语倒装句(Inversions)有两种:完全倒装和部分倒装。倒装是一种语法手段,用于表示一定的句子结构。

一、完全倒装即把整个谓语放到主语之前。

副词位于句首,谓语动词是 be, come, go, follow, run 等表地点、位移的词,主语是名词,用完全倒装。例如:

In came the teacher and the class began.

Here comes the bus.

There appeared to be a man in grey.

Up climbed the girl when her father came.

Out rushed the mad woman.

二、部分倒装即把谓语的一部分,如助动词、be 动词、情态动词等放在主语前。

1. 大部分否定开头的句子用部分倒装形式。例如:

Nor does Henry know the answer.

Neither will Rose go away.

Not until yesterday did Mary make up her mind.

In no country other than Britain can one experience four seasons in a day.

Under no circumstances should you surrender.

Scarcely had they left before soldiers arrived armed with rifles.

2. only 后跟状语，主句用倒装。例如：

Only in an English speaking country can you learn "true English".

3. as 引导的倒装。例如：

Hard as he worked，he failed in the exam.

4. so 引导的倒装。例如：

He promised to fulfill his task. So did I.

So selfish was Tom that no one liked him.

5. 直接引语后面的句子中的主语是名词的需倒装。例如：

"Let's do it," said his mother.

6. 省略 if 的虚拟条件句的倒装。例如：

Were it not for the child，I would not do it.

Should it rain tomorrow，we would postpone the meeting.

7. 感叹句的部分倒装形式。例如：

May you have a magical Christmas!

Practice

1. _____ , I have never seen a more capable man than John.

    A．As long as I have traveled   B．As I travel so much

    C．Now that I have traveled   D．Much as I have traveled

2. So difficult _____ it to live in a foreign country that I decided to leave.

    A．I have felt   B．I did feel

    C．have I felt   D．did I feel

3. Not only _____ to stay at home，but he was also forbidden to see his friends.

    A．He was forcing   B．was he forcing

    C．he was forced   D．was he forced

4. Little _____ about his own health though he was very ill.

    A．he cared   B．does he care

    C．did he care   D．he cares

5. No sooner _____ asleep than she heard a knock at the door.

    A．she had fallen   B．She had fell

    C．had she fallen   D．had she fell

Writing

关于**表格**(Tables)作文，主要注意两点：一是明确表格是用来描述两个或多个事物之间关系的，在作文中要说明上述关系及关系的变化情况；二是掌握描述表格的基本句型。

一、描述表格的基本句型示例

The table describes ...

The table shows the relationship between ... and ...

The table illustrates the changes in ... over the period of ...

There are ... , with ... accounting for the largest ... at... , followed by... at... and ... at...

As is shown in the table, ...

As can be seen from the table, ...

二、部分表示数据变化的表达法

The figures/statistics show (that)...

... were slightly larger/smaller than that of ...

The data/statistics show (that) ...

... peaked(达到顶点) at ... in (month/year)

There was a threefold increase in the number of ...

From then on/From this time onwards ... , ... decreased year by year while ... increased steadily.

The data/statistics/figures lead us to the conclusion that ...

As can be seen from the diagram, great changes have taken place in ...

A is ... times as much/many as B.

A increased by/ to ...

A has something in common with B.

This table shows the changing proportion 比例 from ... to ... .

This table shows high/low/great/small percentages of A & B.

Over the period from ... to ... , the ... remained level/steady/stable/ the same.

In the year between ... and ... , the number sharply went up to ... / bottomed out in ... / be similar to ... / be the same as ...

Practice

Instruction：*Please write a short essay entitled "Flights at Beijing International Airport" based on the following table and outline.*

1. Describe the table below and discuss the problem you can see from it.

2. State your opinion about how to solve the problem.

Beijing International Airport
ARRIVALS

Time	Flight #	Gate	From	Comments
2:10	72	8	Chicago	On time
3:10	117	3	Houston	Landing
4:15	65	6	Boston	Delayed
5:20	711	10	Dallas	Arrived
6:10	80	4	Los Angeles	On time
7:15	76	2	Detroit	On time

Unit Six
Welfare

Guidance

1. This unit consists of Text A, Text B and Further Study. **Text A** tells us about how the American child welfare system works. **Text B** discusses health trends and malnutrition among rural children in China. **Further Study** focuses on communication skills in terms of shopping.

2. By learning this unit, students will be able to master the structure of the texts, new words, phrases and expressions. Students will improve their understanding of grammatical structures, reading comprehension and enlarge their vocabulary by doing the relevant exercises. Meanwhile, they will gain better understanding of different *Welfare* systems.

3. **Further Study** aims to improve students' skills for communication. By doing the exercises, students will know the differences in communication between Chinese and Westerners. They will perform well in everyday conversation and writing by doing this part.

> Sickness is the vengeance of nature for the violation of her laws.
>
> — Charles Simmons

▪▪ Text A How the American Child Welfare System Works

Child Welfare Information Gateway, 2013

The child welfare system is a group of services designed to promote the well-being of children by[1] ensuring safety, achieving permanency, and strengthening families to care for their children successfully. While the primary responsibility for child welfare services rests with the States, the Federal Government plays a major role in supporting States in the delivery of services through funding of programs and legislative initiatives.

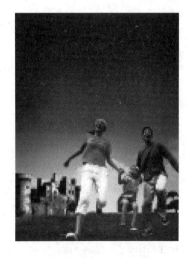

The primary responsibility for implementing Federal child and family legislation rests with the Children's Bureau, within the Administration on Children, Youth and Families, Administration for Children and Families, U.S. Department of Health and Human Services (HHS). The Children's Bureau works with State and local agencies to develop programs that focus on preventing child abuse and neglect by strengthening families, protecting children from further maltreatment, reuniting children safely with their families, or finding permanent families for children who cannot safely return home.

Most families first become involved with their local child welfare system because of a report of suspected child abuse or neglect (sometimes called "child maltreatment"). Child maltreatment is defined by CAPTA as[2] serious harm (neglect, physical abuse, sexual abuse, and emotional abuse or neglect) caused to[3] children by parents or primary caregivers, such as[4] extended family members or babysitters. Child maltreatment also can include harm that a caregiver allows to happen or does not prevent from happening to a child. In general, child welfare agencies do not intervene in cases of harm to children caused by acquaintances or strangers. These cases are the responsibility of law enforcement.

The child welfare system is not a single entity. Many organizations in each community work together to strengthen families and keep children safe. Public agencies, such as departments of social services or child and family services, often contract and collaborate with private child welfare agencies and community-based organizations to provide services to families, such as in-home family preservation services, foster care, residential treatment, mental health care, substance abuse treatment, parenting skills classes, domestic violence services, employment assistance, and financial or housing assistance.

Child welfare systems are complex, and their specific procedures vary widely by State. The purpose of this fact sheet is to give a brief overview of the purposes and functions of child welfare from a national perspective[5]. Child welfare systems typically: receive and investigate reports of possible child abuse and neglect; provide services to families that need assistance in the protection and care of their children; arrange for children to live with kin or with foster families when they are not safe at home; arrange for reunification, adoption, or other permanent family connections for children leaving foster care.

The goal of child welfare is to promote the well-being, permanency, and safety of children and families by helping families care for their children successfully or, when that is not possible, helping children find permanency with kin or adoptive families. Among children who enter foster care, most will return safely to the care of their own families or go to live with relatives or an adoptive family.

New Words

welfare /'welfeə/	*n*. help given, esp. by the state or an organization, to help people who need it, esp. because they do not have enough money 福利救济;社会福利
permanence /'pɜːmənəns/	*n*. staying the same or continuing for a long time 持久(性);永久(性),永恒(性)
federal /'fedərəl/	*adj*. relating to the central government, and not to the government of a region, of some countries such as the United States 联邦政府的
legislative /'ledʒɪslətɪv/	*adj*. relating to laws or the making of laws 法律的;立法的
implement /'ɪmplɪment/	*vt*. to put a plan or system into operation 实施;贯彻
bureau /'bjʊərəʊ/	*n*. a department of government, or a division that performs a particular job (政府部门的)局,处,科
focus /'fəʊkəs/	*n*. the main or central point of something, esp. of attention or interest (尤指注意力或兴趣的)中心,焦点
abuse /ə'bjuːz/	*vt*. to use or treat someone or something wrongly or badly, esp. in a way that is to your own advantage (尤指为个人私利而)虐待,伤害,滥用,妄用
maltreatment /mæl'triːtmənt/	*n*. treating someone cruelly or violently 粗暴对待,虐待
reunite /'riːjuː'naɪt/	*vt*. to bring together again 使重新结合;使再联合;使重聚
suspect /sə'spekt/	*vt*. to think or believe something to be true or probable 怀疑,猜想,认为(某事有可能)
entity /'entɪtɪ/	*n*. something which exists apart from other things, having its own independent existence 实体;独立存在体
contract /kən'trækt/	*v*. to have formally agreed to work for a company or person on a states job for a stated period of time 签订合同(为某公司或某人工作);有合同约束
residential /ˌrezɪ'denʃəl/	*adj*. a position for which you live at the same place where you work or study (为工作或学习而)在某处居住的,寄宿的,住宿在任所的;居住的;定居的
domestic /də'mestɪk/	*adj*. belonging or relating to the home, house or family 家庭的
assistance /ə'sɪstəns/	*n*. help 帮助;协助;援助
perspective /pə'spektɪv/	*n*. a particular way of considering something (思考问题的)角度,观点,想法

Phrases and Expressions

rest with	依靠;依赖;寄托于
legislative initiatives	立法创制权
focus on	集中于;聚焦;专注

defined by ... as...	当作；定义为……
adoptive families	收养家庭

Text Notes

1. by 后接动名词，表示"通过做……"。例如：John accumulated vocabulary by memorizing words every day. 约翰通过每天记单词积累词汇。

2. be defined as 表示"被定义为"。例如：In this dictionary "reality" is defined as "the state of things as they are rather than as they are imagined to be". 在本词典中，"现实"被定义为"事物原本的状态，而非想象的样子"。

3. harm caused to ... 表示"对……引起的伤害"；harm caused by ... 表示"由……引起的伤害"。例如：Actual bodily harm caused by exposure to the sun sometimes goes unnoticed. 暴露在阳光下对身体造成的实际伤害有时未被注意。又如：Actual bodily harm caused to children sometimes goes unnoticed. 对孩子身体造成的实际伤害有时没被注意。

4. such as 表示"诸如"。例如：That sum of money is to cover costs such as travel and accommodation. 那笔钱将包括诸如旅行和住宿的费用。

5. from ... perspective 表示"从……角度"。例如：She writes from a fresh perspective. 她从一个新角度来写。

Text Comprehension

Please choose the best answers to the following questions according to the text.

1. The child welfare system is a group of services designed to promote the well-being of children by _____.
   A. ensuring safety
   B. achieving permanency
   C. strengthening families to care for their children successfully
   D. all of the above

2. What does the word "primary" mean in Para. 2?
   A. Most important.   B. Pertinent.   C. Imminent.   D. Innocent.

3. Which of the following is TRUE according to the passage?
   A. The primary responsibility for implementing Federal child and family legislation rests with U.S. Department of Health and Human Services (HHS) only.
   B. Few families first become involved with their local child welfare system because of a report of suspected child abuse or neglect.
   C. The Children's Bureau works with State and local agencies to develop programs that focus on preventing child abuse and neglect.
   D. Child maltreatment does not include harm that a caregiver allows to happen or does not prevent from happening to a child.

4. Many organizations in each community work together to _____.
   A. strengthen families   B. keep children safe
   C. both A and B   D. None of the above

5. What is the author's purpose of writing this passage?

A. To introduce American child welfare system.

B. To encourage people to protect children from child abuse.

C. To stress the importance of child care.

D. To make an advertisement for some child training centre.

Vocabulary and Structure

Please choose the best answer for each of the following sentences.

1. She is continually _____ her position/authority by getting other people to do things for her.
   A. abusing   B. teasing   C. using   D. tempting

2. This national fund pays for _____ benefits such as unemployment and sickness pay.
   A. fare   B. fair   C. welfare   D. satire

3. A loving family environment gives children that sense of stability and _____ which they need.
   A. exclusion   B. reflection   C. property   D. permanence

4. I don't enjoy _____ activities.
   A. feasible   B. physical   C. sensitive   D. critical

5. She has that reserve and slight coldness of manner which is _____ English.
   A. typically   B. physically   C. economically   D. permanently

Comprehensive Exercise

There are five incomplete sentences in the following passage. Read the passage and choose the word that best fits into the passage. Do remember each word can be used only once.

A. To   B. or   C. per   D. to   E. of

In 2005 China had about 1,938,000 physicians (1.5 per 1,000 persons) and about 3,074,000 hospital beds (2.4 per 1,000 persons). Health expenditures on a purchasing power parity (PPP) basis were US $ 224 __1__ capita in 2001, __2__ 5.5 percent of gross domestic product. Some 37.2 percent of public expenditures were devoted __3__ health care in China in 2001. However, about 80 percent of the health and medical care services are concentrated in cities, and timely medical care is not available to more than 100 million people in rural areas. __4__ offset this imbalance, in 2005 China set out a five-year plan to invest 20 billion Renminbi (RMB; US $ 2.4 billion) to rebuild the rural medical service system composed __5__ village clinics and township- and county-level hospitals.

Translation

Please translate the following sentences into Chinese.

1. He had been badly maltreated as a child.

2. Sarah was finally reunited with her children at the airport.

3. You must satisfy the residential qualifications to get a work permit.

4. Domestic opinion had turned against the war.

5. The company needs more financial assistance from the Government.

∷ Text B   Health Trends and Malnutrition among Rural Children in China

Wikipedia, the free encyclopedia

Since 1949, China had a huge improvement in population's health. In general, all indices show the progresses except the drop around 1960 due to the failure of the Great Leap Forward[1], which led to starvation of 20 million people. As we can see, from 1950 to 2011, life expectancy nearly doubled (41.6~75.0). Total Fertility Rate changed from 5.3 to 1.7 mainly caused by One-Child Policy. Infant Mortality Rate(IMR)[2] and Under 5 Mortality Rate(U5MR)[3]sharply went down. Though there is no data from 1963 to 1967, we can see the trend. The gap between IMR and U5MR became smaller and smaller, which indicates health in children has been promoted. Maternal Mortality Ratio isn't showed in the graph since data insufficiency, but it did go down from 164.5 (1980) to 26.5 (2011).

	1950	1960	1970	1980	1990	2000	2011
Life expectancy	41.6	31.6	62.7	66.1	69.5	72.1	75.0
Total Fertility Rate	5.3	4.3	5.7	2.3	2.5	1.5	1.7
Infant Mortality Rate	195.0	190.0	79.0	47.2	42.2	30.2	12.9
Under 5 Mortality Rate/Child mortality	317.1	309.0	111	61.3	54.0	36.9	14.9
Maternal Mortality Ratio				164.5	88.0	57.5	26.5

China has been developing rapidly for the past 30 years. Though it has uplifted a huge number of people out of poverty, many social issues still remain unsolved. One of them is malnutrition among rural children in China. The problem has diminished but still remains a pertinent national issue. In a survey done in 1998, the stunting rate among children in China was 22 percent and was as high as 46 percent in poor provinces. This shows the huge disparity between urban and rural areas. In 2002, Svedberg found that stunting rate in rural areas of China was 15 percent, reflecting that a substantial number of children still suffer from malnutrition. Another study by Chen shows that malnutrition has dropped from 1990 to 1995 but regional differences are still huge, particularly in rural areas.

In a recent report by The Rural Education Action Project on children in rural China, many were found to be suffering from basic health problems. 34 percent have iron deficiency anaemia and 40 percent are infected with intestinal worms. Many of these children do not have proper or sufficient nutrition. Often, this causes them not being able to fully reap the benefits of education, which can be a ticket out of poverty.

One possible reason for poor nutrition in rural areas is that agricultural produce can fetch a decent price, and thus is often sold rather than kept for personal consumption. Rural families would[4] not consume eggs that their hen lay but will sell it in the market for about 20 yuan per kilogram. The money will then be spent on books or food like instant noodles which lack nutrition value compared to an egg. A girl named Wang Jing in China has a bowl of pork only once every five to six weeks, compared to urban children who have a vast array of food chains to choose from.

A survey conducted by China's Ministry of Health showed the kind of food consumed by rural households. 30 percent consume meat less than once a month. 23 percent consume rice or egg less than[5] once a month. Up to 81 percent consume less than one cup of dairy products a week. Dairy products and eggs provide essential nutrients that are important for a child's physical development.

In a 2008 Report on Chinese Children Nutrition and Health Conditions, West China still has 7.6 million poor children who were shorter and weigh lesser than urban children. These rural children were also shorter by 4 centimeters and 0.6 kilograms lighter than World Health Organization standards. It can be concluded that children in West China still lack quality nutrition.

For China to progress even further, these social issues must be tackled. By uplifting more people out of poverty, more children will also be uplifted out of malnutrition.

New Words

trend /trend/	*n.* a general development or change in a situation or in the way that people are behaving 趋势,趋向;倾向,动向
malnutrition /ˌmælnjuːˈtrɪʃən/	*n.* physical weakness and bad health caused by having too little food, or too little of the types of food necessary for good health 营养不良
rural /ˈrʊərəl/	*adj.* in, of or like the countryside 乡村的,农村的;似乡村的
index /ˈɪndeks/	*n.* ① an alphabetical list, such as one printed at the back of a book showing which page a subject, name, etc. is found on (plural: indexes)(书后关于主题、姓名等的)索引 ② a system of numbers used for comparing values of things that change according to each other or a fixed standard (plural: indices)指数,指标
fertility /fəˈtɪlɪtɪ/	*n.* the quality of being able to produce young or fruit (动植物的)生殖力
infant /ˈɪnfənt/	*n.* a baby or a very young child 婴儿
mortality /mɔːˈtælətɪ/	*n.* The number of deaths within a particular society and within a particular period of time 死亡数量,死亡率
gap /gæp/	*n.* an empty space or opening in the middle of something or between two things 缺口;豁口;裂口
maternal /məˈtɜːnəl/	*adj.* behaving or feeling in the way that a mother does towards her child, esp. in a kind, loving way 母亲的;母亲般的
ratio /ˈreɪʃɪəʊ/	*n.* the relationship between two groups or amounts, which expressed how much bigger one is than the other 比;比例;比率
gragh /grɑːf/	*n.* a picture which shows how two sets of information or various amounts are related, usu. by lines or curves (通常用直线或曲线表示的)图,图表,图解
insufficiency /ˌɪnsəˈfɪʃənsɪ/	*n.* being not enough 不够,不足;不充分

uplift /ˈʌplɪft/	*n.* improvement of a person's moral or spiritual condition（道德境界的）提升,促进;（精神上的）鼓舞,振作
poverty /ˈpɒvətɪ/	*n.* the condition of being extremely poor 贫困,贫穷
pertinent /ˈpɜːtɪnənt/	*adj.* relating directly to the subject being considered 有关的,直接相关的
disparity /dɪˈspærətɪ/	*n.* a state in which there is no equality and similarity, esp. in a way that is not fair; difference 不平等;不等同;差异
deficiency /dɪˈfɪʃənsɪ/	*n.* state of not having, or not having enough, of something that is needed 不足,缺乏,缺少
anaemia /əˈniːmɪə/	*n.* (in AM, use anemia) a medical condition in which there are not enough red blood cells in the blood 贫血（症）
intestinal /ɪnˈtestɪnəl/	*adj.* of a long tube through which food travels from one stomach and out of the body while it is being digested 肠的

Phrases and Expressions

go down	下降
the disparity between ... and ...	……与……之间的不同
drop from ... to ...	从……降至……
reap the benefits of	收获……的果实
a vast array of	（尤指非常有吸引力、令人赞赏并常以特定的方式排列的）一系列,一批,大量,大群

Text Notes

1. the Great Leap Forward 指"大跃进运动"。大跃进运动是指 1958 年至 1960 年间,中国共产党在全国范围内开展的极"左"路线的运动。
2. Infant Mortality Rate (IMR) 表示"婴儿死亡率"。
3. Under 5 Mortality Rate (U5MR) 表示"5 岁以下儿童死亡率"。
4. would 在这里表示一种不太可能实现的假设,是虚拟语气用法。例如:There would be trouble unless the report were finished on time. 除非按时完成报告,否则会有麻烦。
5. less than 表示"更少,较小"。例如:I eat less chocolate and fewer biscuits than I used to. 巧克力和饼干我比以前吃得少了。

Text Comprehension

Please read the following statements and mark T/F according to the text.

1. Since 1949, China had little improvement in population's health.
   A. T   B. F
2. As we can see, from 1950 to 2011, life expectancy in China doubled (41.6~75.0).
   A. T   B. F
3. In a recent report by The Rural Education Action Project on children in rural China, many were found to be suffering from basic health problems.
   A. T   B. F

4. The reason for poor nutrition in rural areas is that agricultural produce can fetch a decent price，and thus is often sold rather than kept for personal consumption.

　　A．T　　　　　　　　　　　B．F

5. Dairy products and eggs provide essential nutrients that are important for a child's physical development.

　　A．T　　　　　　　　　　　B．F

Vocabulary and Structure

Please complete the following sentences with the proper forms of the words given.

1. Many of the refugees are suffering from severe _____ . （nutrition）

2. The chart shows declining _____ rates. （fertile）

3. Her _____ grandmother （mother's mother） is still alive. （maternity）

4. I felt that the whole project was _____ researched. （insufficiency）

5. Pregnant women often suffer from iron _____ . （deficient）

Translation

Please translate the following passage into Chinese.

　　After 1949 the Ministry of Public Health was responsible for all health-care activities and established and supervised all facets of health policy. Along with a system of national，provincial，and local facilities，the ministry regulated a network of industrial and state enterprise hospitals and other facilities covering the health needs of workers of those enterprises. In 1981 this additional network provided approximately 25 percent of the country's total health services.

▪▪ Further Study

（Shopping）

购物（Shopping）：购物时使用的用语很多，掌握主要词语和惯用法是关键。

Key Sentences and Phrases

◆ Questions about shopping
○ How often do you go shopping?
○ Who do you like shopping with?
○ Is the post-sales service of department stores satisfactory?
○ How can a store attract people?
○ What do you think of on-line shopping?
○ Where do you like to do your shopping — in grocery stores，department stores or supermarkets?
◆ Possible answers to questions about shopping
○ I spend most of my weekends shopping.

○ The shop assistants are kind/polite/efficient to give some advice rather than indifferent and arrogant.

○ Goods can be delivered to home.

○ People can order something in advance.

○ It is convenient/saves time and energy to pick up milk or eggs or whatever on my way home from work.

○ Food in the supermarket is clean and not expensive.

○ I sometimes buy things from street vendors.

○ Sitting in front of the computer, one can choose the listed goods by their prices and qualities.

○ Pay through computer and not very long afterwards the goods will be delivered to home.

○ More and more people choose online shopping.

◆ Phrases about shopping

○ go window-shopping

○ get information about fashion

○ one's favorite department store

○ a well-known shopping mall

○ buy fashionable/cute commodities

○ guaranteed with good quality

○ from cosmetics to clothes/jewelries/all brands of appliances

○ find some bargains

○ compulsive shopping

○ do grocery shopping.

○ fake products

○ stand in line

○ in front of the cash register for some time

○ paying the bill

Practice

Please choose the best answer for each of the following sentences.

1. — How do you pay?

   — _____.

   A. By credit card   B. Money   C. Credit   D. Card

2. Please enter your _____ when you pay.

   A. state   B. PIN   C. welfare   D. address

3. — How did you find me selling my dress?

   — I saw your _____.

   A. kite   B. fly   C. book   D. flyer

4. — When do the bids rise most?

   — The bids rise most just before the close of the _____.

   A. auction   B. action   C. activist   D. act

5. — What is a _____ price when the seller sell something online?

   — It is the minimum price the seller can accept.

   A. maximum   B. preserve   C. reserve   D. conserve

Grammar

不定式(Infinitive)：不定式在句子中可作主语、宾语、状语、定语、表语和补足语。不定式的时态：一般式用 to do 或 to be done；完成式用 to have done 或 to have been done；进行式用 to be doing；完成进行式用 to have been doing。此外，注意一些不带 to 的不定式词组的用法。

一、不定式在句子中作主语。

例如：It is necessary for young people to master at least two languages.

It is not easy for you to catch fish barehanded.

It is kind of you to help me with mathematics.

It is a waste of time to read the book.

It takes me three hours to finish the paper.

二、不定式在句子中作宾语。

例如：I'd like to go for a walk in the warm sunshine.

She found it impossible to get everything ready in time.

三、不定式在句子中作定语。

例如：There is no need to bother him with trifles.

His efforts to carry out the plan were successful.

She is a very nice person to work with.

四、不定式在句子中作表语。

例如：My chief purpose is to overcome the difficulties.

His duty is to greet new comers to his school and to provide them with any necessary information.

五、不定式在句子中作补语。

例如：I'd never allow my children to behave like that.

He asked you to call him back.

He saw her mother cry.

The teacher will have the students write a passage.

He is reported to have won the 100 meter race.

Mr. Brown is said to have left for Italy.

六、一些不带 to 的不定式词组的用法。

例如：I would rather not see him.

You'd better return the books on time.

I can't help but pray for them.

They had never seen such food，let alone eat it.

七、不定式在句子中作状语。

例如：They came here to further their studies.

Practice

1. The book is well _____ .

A．worth reading　　B．worthy to read　　C．worth to read　　D．worthy reading

2. Most offices require secretaries _____ .

A．have specified training

B．having specified training

C．to have specified training

D．to have been specified training

3. When _____ remains undecided.

A．to start the program

B．to be starting the program

C．starting the program

D．have started the program

4. It is unwise of you _____ the proposal.

A．turning down

B．turn down

C．having turned down

D．to turn down

5. The room was designed _____ a study.

A．being　　　　　　B．been　　　　　　C．to be　　　　　　D．to have been

Writing

> 柱形图 (Bar Chart, Bar Graph or Column Chart) 是用垂直的柱状图形表示数据的变化, 每根柱子的顶端代表了某方面的数值, 柱子的高低反映了数值的增减变化。

英语柱形图作文基本表达法如下：

The bar chart shows changes in . . . rates.

The most obvious trend in the chart is that . . .

The second biggest trend in the chart is . . .

There is considerable fluctuation in . . .

The numbers increased/fell slightly/markedly/gradually/steadily/ rapidly by 30% . . .

The . . . accounted for 50% of . . .

The number doubled/tripled/quadrupled from . . . to . . .

Practice

Instruction: Please write a short essay entitled *"Unbalanced Development of Mobile Phone Users"* based on the following chart and outline.

1. Describe the chart below and discuss the problem you can see from the chart.

2. State your opinion about how to solve the problem.

Mobile Phone Users per 1,000 People

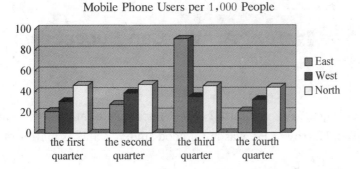

Unit Seven
Great People

- We Can Succeed
- For Blooming in Wards — Nightingale

Guidance

1. This unit consists of Text A, Text B and Further Study. **Text A** tells us the secrets of how to achieve success by the stories of many great people. **Text B** introduces the life story of Nightingale and the great achievements she made to the development of modern hospital. **Further Study** focuses on communication skills.

2. By learning this unit, students will be able to master the structure of the texts, new words, phrases and expressions. Students will improve their understanding of grammatical structures, reading comprehension and enlarge their vocabulary by doing the relevant exercises. Meanwhile, they will get to know the stories of many *Great People*.

3. **Further study** aims to improve students' skills for communication. By doing the exercises, students will know the ways to show agreement and disagreement. They will perform well in everyday conversation and writing by doing this part.

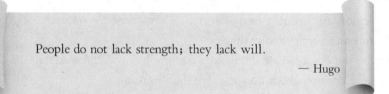

People do not lack strength; they lack will.

— Hugo

▪▪ Text A   We Can Succeed

Anonymous

When Britain's great Prime Minister, Sir Winston Churchill[1], was young, he attended a public school called Harrow[2]. He was not a good student, and as matter of fact, had he not been the son of a famous leader, he probably would have been thrown out of the school for his offences.[3] However, he completed his work at Harrow, went on to the university, and then had a successful career in the British Army, touring both Africa and India. He later was elected prime minister and brought great courage to Britain through his speeches and other work during the dark days of World War II.

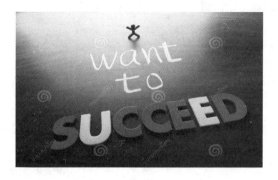

Toward the very end of his period as prime minister, he was invited to address the young boys at his old school, Harrow. In announcing the coming of their great leader[4], the headmaster said, "young gentlemen, the greatest speaker of our time, our prime minister, will be here in a few days to address you, and you should obey whatever sound advice he may give you at that time."

The great day arrived, and the prime minister appeared at Harrow. After being introduced[5], Sir Winston stood up — all five feet, five inches and 107 kilos of him! He gave this short but moving speech: "Young men, never give up. Never give up! Never give up! Never, never, never, never!"

Personal history, education, situation — none of these can hold back a strong spirit. Think, for example, of Abraham Lincoln, who was elected president of the United States in 1860. He grew up on a small farm at what was then the edge of the settled part of the United States. He had only one year of regular education. In those early years, his family hardly had a penny and he only read about half a dozen books. In 1832 he lost his job and was defeated when he tried to get elected to the Illinois government. In 1833 he failed in business. In 1834 he was elected to the state government, but in 1835 the woman he loved died. In 1838 he was defeated when he tried to become a leader in the Illinois government, and in 1843 he was defeated when he tried to enter the U. S. Congress. In 1846 he was elected to Congress but in 1848 lost a second election and was forced out. In 1849 he was refused a job with the national government, and in 1854 he was defeated for the U. S. Senate. In 1856 he was defeated in the election for vice president, and in 1858 he was again defeated for the Senate.

Many people consider Lincoln to be the greatest president of all time. Yet it should be remembered how many failures and defeats marked his early life.

Some of the world's greatest men and women have met huge problems and difficulties at some time in their lives, but have gone on to do great deeds.

Bury him in the snows of Valley Forge, and you have a George Washington.

Make a musical genius unable to hear, and you have a Ludwig van Beethoven.

Have him born black in a society filled with bitter hate between races, and you have a Martin Luther King, Jr.

Call him slow to learn, and write him off as stupid, and you have an Albert Einstein.

New Words

address /əˈdres/   *v.* ① to speak publicly to a group of people 演讲   ② to write the name and address of a particular person or organization on an envelope, package 写地址

      n. the name of the place where you live or work, including the house or office number and the name of the street, area, and town 地址

announce /əˈnaʊns/   *vt. & vi.* to make a public or official statement, especially about a plan, decision, or something that has happened 公布;宣布

attend /əˈtend/   *vt. & vi.* ① to be present at an event or activity 出席;参加   ② to take care of someone, especially someone who is sick or someone in an important position 照顾

bureau /ˈbjʊərəʊ/   *n.* a government department or part of a government department 局;司;署

congress /ˈkɒŋgres/   *n.* the national legislative body of a nation, especially a republic 国会

courage /ˈkʌrɪdʒ/   *n.* the ability to do something that you know is right or good, even though it is dangerous, frightening, or very difficult 勇气;胆量

dozen /ˈdʌzn/   *n.* a set of 12 things or people 十二;一打

edge /edʒ/   *n.* ① the part of something that is farthest from its center 边缘; 外沿   ② the sharp side of a blade or tool that is used for cutting things 刀口;刀刃

fail /feɪl/   *vt. & vi.* ① to be unsuccessful when you try to do something 失败;不成功   ② to not do something that people expect you to do 辜负;有负于

failure /ˈfeɪljə/   *n.* the condition or fact of not achieving the desired end or ends 失败;不成功

federal /ˈfedərəl/   *adj.* of or constituting a form of government in which sovereign power is divided between a central authority and a number of constituent political units 联邦的

focus /ˈfəʊkəs/   *n.* the thing that people are concentrating on or paying particular attention to 关注点;中心;重点

      vt. & vi. to concentrate on something and pay particular attention to it (使)关注;(使)专心于

genius /ˈdʒiːnɪəs/   *n.* someone who is much more intelligent or skillful than other people 天才

government /ˈgʌvənmənt/   *n.* the people who control a country, region, or city and make decisions about its laws and taxes 政府

minister /ˈmɪnɪstə/   *n.* ① a member of government who is in charge of a government department 内阁成员;大臣   ② in some Protestant churches, someone whose job is to lead worship and perform other duties 牧师

offence /əˈfens/	*n.* ① something that you do or say which makes someone else angry or upset 冒犯；触怒 ② a crime or illegal activity for which there is a punishment 进攻；攻击
prime /praɪm/	*adj.* first in excellence, quality, or value 首要的；第一的；主要的
senate /ˈsenət/	*n.* an assembly or a council of citizens having the highest deliberative and legislative functions in a government 参议院
speech /spiːtʃ/	*n.* the faculty or act of expressing or describing thoughts, feelings, or perceptions by the articulation of words 演说；演讲；言辞
spirit /ˈspɪrɪt/	*n.* ① the soul, considered as departing from the body of a person at death 灵魂；精神 ② a particular mood or an emotional state characterized by vigor and animation 活力；生气；志气
tour /tʊə/	*n.* a trip with visits to various places of interest for business, pleasure, or instruction 旅行；旅游；参观；游览
	vt. & vi. to travel from place to place, especially for pleasure 旅行；游览

Phrases and Expressions

as a matter of fact	事实上
be filled with	充满……的；被……填满的
fail in	在……方面失败；在……不及格
grow up	长大；成人
hold back	阻止；阻拦
throw out	驱逐；赶走；扔掉

Text Notes

1. **Winston Churchill**: Sir Winston Leonard Spencer－Churchill(30 November 1874～24 January 1965) was a British politician and Nobel laureate who was the Prime Minister of the United Kingdom from 1940 to 1945 and again from 1951 to 1955. Widely regarded as one of the greatest wartime leaders of the 20th century, Churchill was also an officer in the British Army, a historian, a writer (as Winston S. Churchill), and an artist. Churchill is the only British Prime Minister to have won the Nobel Prize in Literature since its inception in 1901, and was the first person to be made an honorary citizen of the United States.

2. **Harrow**: Harrow School commonly referred to as "Harrow", is an English independent school for boys situated in the town of Harrow, in north-west London. There is some evidence that there has been a school on the site since 1243, but the Harrow School of today was formally founded in 1572 by John Lyon under a Royal Charter of Elizabeth I. Harrow is one of the original nine public schools that were regulated by the Public Schools Act 1868.

3. 句中 had he not been the son of a famous leader 是虚拟条件句"if he had not been the son of a

famous leader"的简略形式。例如：If she had invited me to the party yesterday，I would have gone to. 可以转化成：Had she invited me to the party yesterday，I would have gone to. 如果昨天她邀请我去参加聚会，我会去的。

4. in doing sth. 表示"在做······时"，In announcing the coming of their great leader 相当于 When announcing the coming of their great leader，可看做时间状语。例如：In handing down the paper，our teacher told us we had thirty minutes to finish it. 发卷子时，老师告诉我们要在三十分钟内完成。

5. After being introduced：以 when，while 等引导的时间状语从句和以 if 引导的条件状语从句，谓语动词是主动语态时，如果从句谓语动词所表示的动作是与主句谓语同时发生，可简化为现在分词的一般式。例如：Before we do the job(= Before doing the job)，we'd better think it over. 在做这项工作之前，我们最好仔细想一想。

Text Comprehension

Please choose the best answers to the following questions according to the text.

1. Which of the following statement is not true according to the article?
   A. Winston Churchill was not a good student when he studied at Harrow.
   B. Winston Churchill had been thrown out of school because of his bad behavior.
   C. Winston Churchill was considered the greatest speaker in his time.
   D. Winston Churchill's speech filled great courage to British people.

2. Which can be inferred from the article?
   A. Winston Churchill did not like to give speech at Harrow.
   B. Winston Churchill was very busy.
   C. Winston Churchill did not prepare the speech carefully.
   D. Winston Churchill intended to encourage the young people to stick to their believes.

3. What does Lincoln's story tell us?
   A. It is hard for child from poor family to succeed.
   B. People's personal experience may prevent their wishes coming true.
   C. People should never give up their dreams.
   D. Success can come only after many failures.

4. Which statement is true according to the article?
   A. Lincoln came from a rich family.
   B. Lincoln was well-educated when he was young.
   C. Lincoln read widely in his childhood.
   D. Lincoln experienced many hardships before he was elected president.

5. What did the author want to tell us by giving the examples of Washington and Beethoven，etc. ？
   A. The author wants to show there are many people experienced more hardships than Lincoln.
   B. The author wants to show great people never give up to hardships in life.
   C. Lincoln was not the only great people in the world.
   D. In different fields there are great people.

Vocabulary and Structure

Please choose the best answer for each of the following sentences.

1. After _____ on the trousers, he found they were 2 inches too long.

   A. putting   B. put

   C. to put   D. being put

2. This is not the correct way to _____ the audience.

   A. talk   B. address

   C. say   D. chat

3. Had I got there five minutes earlier, I could _____ her.

   A. meet   B. meeting

   C. have met   D. to meet

4. It is his first visit to Europe as the _____.

   A. preside   B. resident

   C. presidency   D. president

5. He grew _____ in a small village in North China.

   A. out   B. down

   C. up   D. on

Comprehensive Exercise

There are five incomplete sentences in the following passage. Read the passage and choose the word that best fits into the passage. Do remember each word can be used only once.

| A. finally | B. sneak | C. on | D. practicing | E. so |

It was soon clear I couldn't stay in China forever. To become a world-class musician, I had to play __1__ the world's big stages. So in 1997, my father and I moved again, this time to Philadelphia, __2__ I could attend the Curtis Institute of Music. __3__ our money worries were easing. The school paid for an apartment and even lent me a Steinway (斯坦威钢琴). At night, I would __4__ into the living room just to touch the keys.

Now that I was in America, I wanted to become famous, but my new teachers reminded me that I had a lot to learn. I spent two years __5__, and by 1999 I had worked hard enough for fortune to take over. The Chicago Symphony orchestra heard me play and liked me, but orchestra schedules were set far in advance. I thought I might join them in a few years.

Translation

Please translate the following sentences into Chinese.

1. As a matter of fact, he is several inches taller than his father.

2. In entering the room, he found he had forgotten his book.

3. They could do nothing to hold back the enemy's attack.

4. I failed in math exam last semester.

5. The hospital is filled with people suffering flu.

■■ Text B   For Blooming in Wards — Nightingale

Anonymous

In May 1857 a Commission to study the whole question of the army medical service began to sit. The price was high. Florence Nightingale[1] was doing this tough work because it was vital, not because she had chosen it.

That summer of 1857 was a nightmare for Florence — not only was she working day and night to deal with the people in the Commission, she was writing her own confidential report about her experiences.

It took Florence only six months to complete her own one-thousand-page Confidential Report, Notes on Matters Affecting the Health, Efficiency and Hospital Administration of the British Army. It was an incredibly clear, deeply-considered work. Every single thing she had learned from Crimea was there — every statement she made was backed by hard evidence.

Florence Nightingale was arguing for prevention rather than cure. It was a new idea then and many politicians and army medical men felt it was revolutionary and positively strange. They firmly opposed Florence and her allies.

She was forced to prove that the soldiers were dying because of their basic living conditions. She had checked dozens of hospitals and barracks and now exposed them as damp, dirty and unventilated. She showed that the soldiers' diet was poor. She collected statistics which proved that the death rate for young soldiers in peace time was double that of the normal population.[2]

She showed that, though the army took only the fittest young men, every year 1,500 were killed by neglect, poor food and disease. She declared "our soldiers enlist to death in the barracks", and this became the battle cry of her supporters.

The hard work on the Commission was now over, but Florence was to continue studying, planning and pressing[3] for army medical reform for the next thirty years.

People now began to demand that she apply her knowledge to civilian hospitals, which she found to be "just as bad or worse" than military hospitals. In 1859 she published a book called Notes on Hospitals. It showed the world why people feared to be taken into hospitals and how matters could be treated.

Florence set forth the then revolutionary theory that[4] simply by improving the construction and physical maintenance, hospital deaths could be greatly reduced. More windows, better ventilation, improved drainage, less crowded conditions, and regular cleaning of the floors, walls and bed frames were basic measures that every hospital could take.

Florence soon became an expert on the building of hospitals and all over the world hospitals were established according to her plan. She wrote hundreds and hundreds of letters from her sofa in London inquiring about sinks and saucepans, locks and laundry rooms. No detail was too small for her considered attention. She worked out ideas for the most efficient way to distribute clean linen, the best method of keeping food hot, the correct number of inches between beds.⁵ She intended to change the administration of hospitals from top to toe. Lives depended upon detail.

Florence Nightingale succeeded. All over the world Nightingale-style hospitals would be built. And Florence would continue to advise on hospital plans for over forty years. Today's hospitals with their flowers and bright, clean and cheerful wards are a direct result of her work.

New Words

administration /ədˌmɪnɪˈstreɪʃn/	*n*. the activities involved in managing a business, organization, or institution 管理;支配
ally /ˈælaɪ/	*n*. someone who is ready to help you, especially against someone else who is causing problems for you 伙伴;盟友
barrack /ˈbærək/	*n*. a building or group of buildings used to house military personnel 兵营;营房
bloom /bluːm/	*n*. ① the flower of a plant 花 ② a condition or time of vigor, freshness, and beauty; prime 全盛期;茂盛时期
	vt. & *vi*. ① to bear a flower or flowers 开花 ② to develop successfully, or to become more healthy and attractive 变得健康或快乐自信
civilian /səˈvɪlɪən/	*n*. a person following the pursuits of civil life, especially one who is not an active member of the military or the police 平民;百姓
commission /kəˈmɪʃn/	*n*. ① a group of people that is officially put in charge of something or asked to find out about something 委员会 ② an extra amount of money that you have to pay to a bank or other organization when they provide a service for you 代办手续费;佣金
confidential /ˌkɒnfɪˈdenʃəl/	*adj*. ① showing that what you are going to say must be kept secret 保密的 ② entrusted with the confidence of another 极信任的;心腹的
double /ˈdʌbl/	*n*. twice as much, or twice as many 两倍
	vt. & *vi*. to become twice as big, twice as much, or twice as many (使)变成两倍
drainage /ˈdreɪnɪdʒ/	*n*. ① the process of taking away water or waste liquid from somewhere 排水;泄水 ② a system of pipes and passages that take away water or waste liquid from an area 排水系统
efficiency /ɪˈfɪʃnsɪ/	*n*. the ability to work well and produce good results by using the available time, money, supplies, etc. 效率;功效
enlist /ɪnˈlɪst/	*vt*. & *vi*. ① to engage (persons or a person) for service in the armed forces 使入伍;使参军 ② to enter the armed forces 入伍;参军
evidence /ˈevɪdəns/	*n*. facts or physical signs that help to prove something 根据;理由
expose /ɪkˈspəʊz/	*vt*. & *vi*. ① to fail to protect someone or something from something

harmful or dangerous 袒露；裸露　② to allow something that is usually covered or hidden to be seen 公布；公开

incredibly /ɪnˈkredəblɪ/   *adv*. beyond belief or understanding；unbelievable 难以置信地

laundry /ˈlɔːndrɪ/   *n*. ① dirty clothes that you are washing, or clean clothes that have just been washed 已洗熨好的衣物；待洗熨的衣物　② a business that washes and irons clothes 洗衣房；洗衣店

linen /ˈlɪnɪn/   *n*. light cloth made from a plant called flax 亚麻布；亚麻纱

maintenance /ˈmeɪntənəns/   *n*. work that is done to keep something such as a building, machine, or piece of equipment repaired and in good condition 保养；维护；维持

nightmare /ˈnaɪtmeə/   *n*. a very frightening and unpleasant dream 噩梦；梦魇

press /pres/   *vt*. & *vi*. ① to push one thing against another 按；压；挤　② to try in a determined way to make someone do something or tell you something 敦促；催促；督促

revolutionary /ˌrevəˈluːʃənərɪ/   *adj*. new and completely changing the way that something is done, thought about, or made 革新的；突破的

saucepan /ˈsɔːspən/   *n*. a round deep metal container with a long handle, used for cooking food on a stove 有柄的深平底祸

statement /ˈsteɪtmənt/   *n*. a written or spoken announcement on an important subject that someone makes in public 声明；说明；陈述

statistics /stəˈtɪstɪks/   *n*. the mathematics of the collection, organization, and interpretation of numerical data, especially the analysis of population characteristics by inference from sampling 统计资料；统计数据

unventilated /ʌnˈventɪleɪtɪd/   *adj*. not ventilated 不通风的

Phrases and Expressions

day and night   夜以继日地；日日夜夜
press for   敦促；迫切要求
rather than   与其……不如……
set forth   公布；宣布；提出

Text Notes

1. **Florence Nightingale**：(12 May 1820～13 August 1910) was a celebrated English social reformer and statistician，and the founder of modern nursing. She came to prominence while serving as a nurse during the Crimean War，where she tended to wounded soldiers. She was known as "the Lady with the Lamp" after her habit of making rounds at night.

2. 通常说"增加了……倍"，不包括基数，即纯增加。若说"增加到……倍"或"是原来的……倍"，则包括基数。例如：This river is as wide again as that river. 这条河的宽度是那条河的 2 倍(这条河比那条河宽 1 倍)。They have produced four fold as many washers as they did last year. 他们今年生产的洗衣机相当于去年的 4 倍。... the death rate for young soldiers in peace time was double that of the normal population：此从句中"that"指代的是前面提到的 the death rate，这种

替代是为了避免表达上的重复。例如：The size of the newly broadened square is four times that of the previous one. 重新拓宽的广场是先前广场的四倍。

3. 此句中，continue studying 表示接着学习。如果上下文并没有明确指出是接着做不同的事，还是接着做同一件事，只说接着做，继续做，那么 continue doing 和 continue to do 可以互换。但有时 continue to do 表示继续做另一件事情（已经完成一件工作）。例如：After he finished reading a novel, he continued to play games with his friends. 他读完小说后跟朋友们继续玩游戏。

4. 这里 that 引导的是同位语从句，详细说明前面 theory 所指代的内容。类似的表达还有：the report that，the saying that，the remark that 等。例如：We heard the news that our team had won. 我们听到消息说我们队赢了。

5. 此句中 the most efficient way to distribute clean linen，the best method of keeping food hot 和 the correct number of inches between beds 都是 for 的宾语。本句可译为：她想出最有效发放干净的被褥以及最好的保温食物的方法，算出床与床之间最恰当的距离。

Text Comprehension

Please read the following statements and mark T/F according to the text.

1. The summer of 1857 was hard for Nightingale because she had too many tasks to do.

   A. T   B. F

2. Nightingale's Confidential Report is about factors affecting health, efficiency and hospital administration in civilian hospital.

   A. T   B. F

3. For Nightingale prevention and cure are equally important.

   A. T   B. F

4. Nightingale's idea was considered new and got support from army medical men.

   A. T   B. F

5. Death rate in war time is higher than peace time.

   A. T   B. F

Vocabulary and Structure

Please complete the following sentences with the proper forms of the words given.

1. She could not bear to live in a _____ room. （ventilate）
2. This _____ ruined his reputation by accepting bribes. （politics）
3. The president has decreed that all males will have to _____. （list）
4. Every day I really have to battle to get on the bus, it's always so _____. （crowd）
5. My house has a _____ system that will not be fouled up by large quantities of refuse. （drain）

Translation

Please translate the following passage into Chinese.

Florence set forth the then revolutionary theory that simply by improving the construction and physical maintenance, hospital deaths could be greatly reduced. She soon became an expert on the building of hospitals and all over the world hospitals were established according to her plan. Florence Nightingale succeeded. All over the world Nightingale-style hospitals would be built.

■ Further Study

（Agreement and Disagreement）

Communication Skills

同意和反对(Agreement and Disagreement)：赞成还是反对,这是我们在日常生活中经常要回答的问题。人们对各种事物的看法与见解往往千差万别；对于同一事物,因为观察者所处的立场或观察的角度不同,得出的结论也往往迥然相异。我们要学会尊重现实,对具体的事物,既要善于表达自己赞成与否,同时要充分尊重别人的意见。

Key Sentences

◆ Agreement
○ There is no doubt about it that...
○ I completely / absolutely agree with you.
○ I agree with you entirely.
○ I totally agree with you.
○ I simply must agree with that.
○ I am of the same opinion.
○ That's exactly what I think.
◆ Disagreement
○ I don't agree with you.
○ I'm sorry, but I disagree.
○ I'm afraid, I can't agree with you.
○ The problem is that...
○ I (very much) doubt whether...
○ This is in complete contradiction to...
○ I am of a different opinion because...
○ I cannot share this / that / the view.
○ I cannot agree with this idea.
○ What I object to is...
○ I have my own thoughts about that.

Practice

1. — I think the shop is closed at this time of day.
   — _____

   A. No, I think it's open.   B. No, I think it's closed.

C. Yes，I think it's open.　　　　　　　D. Yes，I don't think so.

2. — I think foreign languages are more interesting than science.

— _____

A. I totally agree with you. I prefer science.

B. I really can't agree with you. I prefer science.

C. I am of a different opinion because I like foreign languages very much.

D. I completely agree with you. I love science，too.

3. — I think I shall read a book instead.

— _____

A. Great. Watching TV programme is much better.

B. No way. Our TV set doesn't work now.

C. OK. Let's turn on the TV set.

D. Good idea. That's much better than watching a bad TV programme.

4. — I don't think that it's true. He's always telling strange stories.

— _____

A. Why not!

B. I am of the same opinion. I think his story is true this time.

C. I know. But this time I can't decide if he is right or not.

D. I cannot share your view. It must be a false story.

5. — Don't think in Chinese when you're speaking English.

— _____

A. You are quite right. I just think in Chinese.　　B. I'm sorry，but I think in English.

C. You can say that again.　　　　　　　　　　　D. It's nonsense.

Grammar

> 主谓一致(Subject-Verb Concord)：主谓一致指句子的主语和谓语动词在人称和数形式上的一致关系。

分类	意义	例句
语法一致原则	句子主语和谓语动词在单复数形式上保持一致	He likes skating in winter. 他喜欢冬天滑冰
意义一致原则	句子主语和谓语动词的一致关系并非取决于主语的单复数形式，而是取决于主语的单复数意义	His family were watching TV when I got to his home. 我到他家时，他家的人在看电视
就近原则	当句子中有若干个并列主语出现，谓语动词的单复数形式由最靠近它的名词决定	There is a desk and five chairs in his room. 他房间里有一张办公桌和五把椅子　There are five chairs and a desk in his room. 他房间里有五把椅子和一张办公桌

Practice

1. Neither he nor I _____ for the plan.
   A. were   B. is   C. are   D. am

2. Twenty miles _____ a long way to cover.
   A. seem to be   B. is   C. are   D. were

3. The students in our school each _____ an English dictionary.
   A. are having   B. had   C. has   D. have

4. Who _____ the girl singing in the next room? Who _____ these people over there?
   A. are; are   B. are; is   C. is; are   D. is; is

5. The population of the earth _____ increasing fast. One third of the population here _____ workers.
   A. is; are   B. is; is   C. are; is   D. are; are

Writing

曲线图(Line Graph)：曲线图是动态图，解题的切入点在于描述趋势。

1. 在开头部分对整个曲线进行一个阶段式的总分类，使写作层次清晰。接下来再分类描述每个阶段的趋势说明，同时导入数据作为分类的依据。

2. 趋势说明 specific trend。即对曲线的连续变化进行说明，如上升、下降、波动、持平。以时间为比较基础的应抓住"变化"：上升、下降、波动。题中对两个或两个以上的变量进行描述时应在此基础上进行比较，如变量多于两个应进行分类或有侧重的比较。

3. 极点说明。即对图表中最高的、最低的点单独进行说明。不以时间为比较基础的应注意对极点的描述。

Practice

Instructions：下面的曲线图是我国2006年不同月份汽车事故分布示意图，请以"*The Number of Car Accidents in 2006*"为题写一篇文章。要求：

1. 描述不同月份汽车事故分布(distribution)及总趋势。
2. 描述汽车事故的可能原因和对策。
3. 参考词汇：peak 顶点，高峰。词数：100～120 。

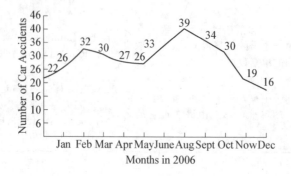

Unit Eight
Science

Guidance

1. This unit consists of Text A, Text B and Further Study. **Text A** tells us the wonder of people about life on other planets. **Text B** reveals that learning can rewire the brain. **Further Study** focuses on communication skills.

2. By learning this unit, students will be able to master the structure of the texts, new words, phrases and expressions. Students will improve their understanding of grammatical structures, reading comprehension and enlarge their vocabulary by doing the relevant exercises. Meanwhile, they will gain better understanding on *Science*.

3. **Further Study** aims to improve students' skills for communication. By doing the exercises, students will know the differences in communication between Chinese and Westerners. They will perform well in everyday conversation and writing by doing this part.

- About Life on Other Planets
- Learning Rewires the Brain

The most beautiful thing we can experience is the mysterious. It is the source of all true art and science.
— Albert Einstein

▋▋ Text A About Life on Other Planets

Darlene Zagata

Humankind continues to wonder whether we are truly alone in the cosmic scheme of existence. People have looked to the heavens throughout the ages and wondered if there is

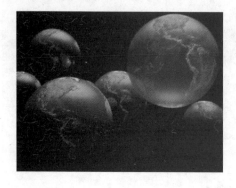

life on other planets. It only seems reasonable there would be some form of life elsewhere, although that life may be in forms we would not even recognize as life — at least not in the intelligent, sentient sense.

History

Since the discovery of other planets in our own solar system, people have wondered about life on other planets. For the longest time, scientists speculated that there may be life on Mars since it is similar to Earth in many ways, but we still seem to be the only life in our solar system. It would be possible for life to develop on other Earth-like planets[1] and moons, but there are many factors to consider such as temperature and the existence of water, as[2] water is an important component in the development of life.

Features

Earth is a planet composed of rock and metal. Along with water, all life on Earth requires oxygen, carbon, phosphorus, nitrogen and hydrogen. We are often referred to as carbon-based life forms[3]. It is believed that these basic materials would be needed for the emergence of life elsewhere in the universe but some scientists argue otherwise, suggesting that life could form from different elements and materials[4]. It has been suggested that there could be silicon-based life forms[5] rather than carbon based. It is possible that different constituents under varying conditions could produce life forms rather different than our own.

Types

Life on Earth shows a wide diversity in forms, yet many contain basic similarities. The same possibility could hold true about life elsewhere in the universe. Life forms could be humanoid and similar to our own or they could be vastly different. The search for other Earth-like planets has led to the discovery of several extra solar planetary bodies in recent years, but most of them are gas giants.

Significance

The human imagination can be quite creative when trying to imagine what other life forms would look like. We've seen numerous examples of this in movies and television shows.

Effects

Life is an ongoing process so it seems probable that life exists elsewhere in the universe in a multitude of different forms and stages of progression. Just as it is possible that life exists elsewhere in forms similar to the bacteria and viruses found on Earth, it is also likely that life forms may exist that are more advanced than humans. Even though many planets have harsh conditions in which life as we know it would not be able to exist, we should keep in mind that there are many creatures on Earth that can exist in harsh climatic conditions. Life could exist in the smallest organic molecules or in a form completely unknown to humanity that could go totally unrecognized. We assume that life could not exist on the giant gaseous planets, but it could very well be possible that some form of life completely beyond the scope of our imaginations may exist.

Considerations

We don't know whether life in any form exists on other planets elsewhere in the universe. Although we have made great strides in our search for extraterrestrial life and the exploration of space our technology is still in its infancy in the cosmic scheme of things. We have barely begun to scratch the surface of galactic exploration. The universe is vast and the number of planets may be immeasurable，at least by our current standards.

New Words

humankind /ˌhjuːmənˈkaɪnd/	*n*. people in general（统称）人；人类
cosmic /ˈkɒzmɪk/	*adj*. ① connected with the whole universe 宇宙的　② very great and important 巨大且重要的
scheme /skiːm/	*n*. a plan or system for doing or organizing sth. 计划；方案；体系；体制
existence /ɪɡˈzɪst(ə)ns/	*n*. the state or fact of being real or living or of being present 存在；实有
intelligent /ɪnˈtelɪdʒ(ə)nt/	*adj*. ① good at learning, understanding and thinking in a logical way about things; showing this ability 有才智的；悟性强的；聪明的　② able to understand and learn things 有智力的；有理解和学习能力的　③ able to store information and use it in new situations 智能的
sentient /ˈsentɪənt/	*adj*. able to see or feel things through the senses 有感觉能力的；有知觉力的
solar /ˈsəʊlə(r)/	*adj*. ① of or connected with the sun 太阳的　② using the sun's energy 太阳能的
speculate /ˈspekjʊleɪt/	*vi*. to form an opinion about sth. without knowing all the details or facts 推测；猜测；推断
oxygen /ˈɒksɪdʒ(ə)n/	*n*. a nonmetallic bivalent element that is normally a colorless odorless tasteless nonflammable diatomic gas 氧；氧气
carbon /ˈkɑː(r)bən/	*n*. a chemical element found in all living things, existing in a pure state as diamond, graphite and buckminsterfullerene 碳
phosphorus /ˈfɒsfərəs/	*n*. a chemical element found in several different forms, including as a poisonous, pale yellow substance that shines in the dark and starts to burn as soon as it is placed in air 磷
nitrogen /ˈnaɪtrədʒ(ə)n/	*n*. a common nonmetallic element that is normally a colorless odorless tasteless inert diatomic gas 氮；氮气
constituent /kənˈstɪtjʊənt/	*n*. one of the parts of sth. that combine to form the whole 成分；构成要素
ongoing /ˈɒnˌɡəʊɪŋ/	*adj*. continuing to exist or develop 持续存在的；仍在进行的；不断发展的
multitude /ˈmʌltɪˌtjuːd/	*n*. ① an extremely large number of things or people 众多；大量

② the mass of ordinary people 群众;大批百姓;民众　③ a large crowd of people 人群

progression /prəʊˈgreʃ(ə)n/　*n*. ① the process of developing gradually from one stage or state to another (进入另一阶段的)发展;前进;进程　② a number of things that come in a series 系列;序列;连续

bacteria /bækˈtɪərɪə/　*n*. /pl/ the simplest and smallest forms of life which exist in large numbers in air, water and soil, and also in living and dead creatures and plants, and are often a cause of disease 细菌

virus /ˈvaɪrəs/　*n*. ① a living thing, too small to be seen without a microscope, that causes infectious disease in people, animals and plants 病毒　② instructions that are hidden within a computer program and are designed to cause faults or destroy data (计算机程序中的)病毒

harsh /hɑː(r)ʃ/　*adj*. ① cruel, severe and unkind 残酷的;严酷的;严厉的　② very difficult and unpleasant to live in 恶劣的　③ too strong and bright; ugly or unpleasant to look at 强烈刺眼的;丑陋的　④ too strong and rough and likely to damage sth. 粗糙的;毛糙的;刺激性强的

creature /ˈkriːtʃə(r)/　*n*. ① a living thing, real or imaginary, that can move around, such as an animal 生物;动物　② a person, considered in a particular way (具有某种特征的)人

climatic /klaɪˈmætɪk/　*adj*. of or relating to a climate 气候的

organic /ɔː(r)ˈgænɪk/　*adj*. ① produced or practised without using artificial chemicals 有机的;不使用化肥的;绿色的　② produced by or from living things 有机物的;生物的　③ connected with the organs of the body 器官的;器质性的

humanity /hjuːˈmænətɪ/　*n*. ① people in general (统称)人;人类　② the state of being a person rather than a god, an animal or a machine 人性　③ the quality of being kind to people and animals by making sure that they do not suffer more than is necessary; the quality of being humane 人道;仁慈

unrecognized /ʌnˈrekəgnaɪzd/　*adj*. ① that people are not aware of or do not realize is important 未被意识到的;被忽略的;不受重视的　② not having received the admiration they deserve for sth. that they have done or achieved 被埋没的;未得到赏识的

gaseous /ˈgeɪsɪəs/　*adj*. like or containing gas 似气体的;含气体的

stride /straɪd/　*n*. ① one long step; the distance covered by a step 大步;一步(的距离)　② your way of walking or running 步态;步伐　③ an improvement in the way sth. is developing 进展;进步;发展

extraterrestrial /ˌekstrətəˈrestrɪəl/　*adj*. connected with life existing outside the planet Earth 地球外的;外星球的;宇宙的

n. (in stories) a creature that comes from another planet; a creature that may exist on another planet（故事中的）天外来客，外星人，外星生物

infancy /ˈɪnfənsɪ/	*n*. ① the time when a child is a baby or very young 婴儿期；幼儿期 ② the early development of sth. 初期；初创期
barely /ˈbeə(r)lɪ/	*adv*. ① in a way that is just possible but only with difficulty 仅仅；刚刚；勉强可能 ② in a way that almost does not happen or exist 几乎不；几乎没有 ③ just；certainly not more than（a particular amount，age，time，etc.）刚好；不超过（某个数量、年龄、时间等）
scratch /skrætʃ/	*vt*. to rub your skin with your nails, usually because it is itching 挠，搔（痒处）
galactic /gəˈlæktɪk/	*n*. relating to a galaxy 银河的；星系的

Phrases and Expressions

be composed of	由……组成
keep in mind	记住
in search for	追求；搜寻；探求
at least	至少

Text Notes

1. Earth-like planets 意为"类地行星"。
2. 此处 as 为连词，表示"因为，由于"。例如：I was worried，as she was as white as a sheet. 我很担心，因为她面色苍白。
3. carbon-based life forms 意为"碳基生物"。
4. suggesting that life could form from different elements and materials 为伴随状语，由于逻辑主语 some scientists 是 suggest 这一动作的主动实施者，故 suggest 用 ing 形式，如果逻辑主语是动作的被动承受者，则分词用 ed 形式。例如：He came in, followed by his wife. 他走了进来，后面跟着他的妻子。
5. silicon-based life forms 意为"硅基生命形式"。

Text Comprehension

Please choose the best answers to the following questions according to the text.

1. The scientists speculated that there may be life on Mars _____ .
   A. because of its temperature
   B. because of the existence of water on it
   C. because of its thin atmosphere
   D. because it is similar to Earth in many ways
2. What does the word "diversity" mean in Para. 4?
   A. Similarity.　　　B. Variety.　　　C. Possibility.　　　D. Change.
3. Which sentence is NOT true according to the passage?
   A. It seems possible that life exists elsewhere in the universe.

　　B．It is likely that there are life forms which are more advanced than humans.

　　C．There can't be lives elsewhere in the universe because many planets have harsh conditions.

　　D．There are much to be explored and found for the galactic exploration.

4. What does the expression "in its infancy" mean in Para. 7?

　　A．Becoming an infant.　　　　　　　B．At young age.

　　C．In the process of growing up.　　　　D．In the initial stage.

5. What's the author's attitude towards the possibility of life on other planets?

　　A．Positive.　　　　B．Negative.　　　　C．Neutral.　　　　D．Indifferent.

Vocabulary and Structure

Please choose the best answer for each of the following sentences.

1. Make sure this meat cooks for _____ an hour.

　　A．at large　　　　　　　　　　　B．in any case

　　C．at least　　　　　　　　　　　D．at last

2. He said he would be poor _____ get money in such a dishonest way.

　　A．in order to　　　　　　　　　　B．instead of

　　C．than　　　　　　　　　　　　D．rather than

3. An _____ computer will be an indispensable diagnostic tool for doctors.

　　A．essential　　　　　　　　　　B．smart

　　C．intelligent　　　　　　　　　　D．sentient

4. _____ more time，we could have done it better.

　　A．Given　　　　　　　　　　　B．Having given

　　C．Giving　　　　　　　　　　　D．Being given

5. _____ it is raining，you'd better take a taxi.

　　A．If　　　　　　B．Provided　　　　C．Due to　　　　D．As

Comprehensive Exercise

There are five incomplete sentences in the following passage. Read the passage and choose the word that best fits into the passage. Do remember each word can be used only once.

A．like	B．in	C．around	D．to	E．toward

　　When it comes __1__ gravity，the larger an object is，the stronger its force is. A person creates gravity but not enough to pull objects __2__ him or cause things to go into orbit __3__ him. On the other hand，a planet has enough gravity to pull objects into orbit around it. A star makes enough gravity that it can pull whole solar systems into its orbit，__4__ ours. Our sun's gravity is so strong that it keeps an object — Pluto — that is roughly 3.7 billion miles away __5__ orbit.

Translation

Please translate the following sentences into Chinese.

1. There is an ongoing debate on the issue.

2. The houses in my hometown were chiefly composed of wood.

3. The professor walked out of the hall, followed by his assistants.

4. Not knowing his address, I can't write to him.

5. He was unrecognized in his disguise.

■■ Text B   Learning Rewires the Brain

Alison Pearce Stevens

Musicians, athletes and quiz bowl[1] champions all have one thing in common: training. Learning to play an instrument or a sport requires time and patience. It is all about steadily mastering new skills. The same is true when it comes to learning information — preparing for that quiz bowl, say, or studying for a big test.

As teachers, coaches and parents everywhere like to say: Practice makes perfect[2].

Doing something over and over again doesn't just make it easier. It actually changes the brain. That may not come as a surprise. But exactly how that process happens has long been a mystery. Scientists have known that the brain continues to develop through our teenage years. But these experts used to think that those changes stopped once the brain matured.

No more.[3]

Recent data have been showing that the brain continues to change over the course of our lives. Cells grow. They form connections with new cells. Some stop talking to others. And it's not just nerve cells that shift and change as we learn. Other brain cells also get into the act.

Scientists have begun unlocking these secrets of how we learn, not only in huge blocks of tissue, but even within individual cells.

Cells that fire together, wire together

Spreng's findings involve the whole brain. However, those changes actually reflect what's happening at the level of individual cells.

The brain is made up of billions of nerve cells, called neurons. These cells are chatty. They "talk" to each other, mostly using chemical messengers. Incoming signals cause a listening neuron to fire or send signals of its own. A cell fires when an electrical signal travels through it. The signal moves away from what is called the cell body, down through a long structure called an axon. When the signal reaches the end of the axon, it triggers the release of those chemical messengers. The chemicals then leap across a tiny gap. This triggers the next cell to fire. And on it goes.

As we learn something new, cells that send and receive information about the task become more and more efficient. It takes less effort for them to signal the next cell about what's going on. In a sense, the neurons become wired together.

Spreng detected that wiring. As cells in a brain area related to some task became more efficient, they used less energy to chat. This allowed more neurons in the "daydreaming" region of the brain to rev up their activity.

Neurons can signal to several neighbors at once. For example，one neuron might transmit information about the location of a baseball pitch that's flying toward you. Meanwhile，other neurons alert your muscles to get ready to swing the bat. When those neurons fire at the same time，connections between them strengthen. That improves your ability to connect with the ball.

Bergstrom stresses the importance of sleep in forming the new memories needed to gain knowledge.[4] So the next time you study for a test，start learning new information a few days ahead of time. The night before，give your brain a break and go to bed early. It will allow your brain a chance to cement that new information into its cells. And that should boost your chances of doing well.

New Words

rewire /rɪˈwaɪr/   *vt*. to provide with new wiring 重新接线；再接电线

steadily /ˈstɛdəlɪ/   *adv*. at a steady rate or pace 稳定地

nerve /nɜː(r)v/   *n*. any of the long threads that carry messages between the brain and parts of the body, enabling you to move，feel pain, etc. 神经

unlock /ʌnˈlɒk/   *vt*. ① to undo the lock of a door，window，etc.，using a key（用钥匙）开……的锁 ② to discover sth. and let it be known 发现；揭示；揭开

tissue /ˈtɪsjuː/   *n*. ① a collection of cells that form the different parts of humans，animals and plants（人、动植物细胞的）组织 ② a piece of soft paper that absorbs liquids，used especially as a handkerchief（尤指用作手帕的）纸巾，手巾纸

fire /ˈfaɪə(r)/   *vt*. & *vi*. ① to start firing a weapon 开火 ② to drive out or away by or as if by fire（以某种燃料）驱动 ③ to terminate the employment of 解雇
   n. ① the flames，light and heat，and often smoke，that are produced when sth. burns 火 ② an occurrence of uncontrolled burning which destroys buildings，forests，or other things 火灾；失火

wire /waɪr/   *vt*. to provide with electrical circuits 给……布线
   n. ① a long thin piece of metal that is used to fasten things or to carry electric curren 金属丝；金属线 ② a cable which carries power or signals from one place to another 电线；导线；电缆

neuron /ˈnjʊərɒn/   *n*. a cell that carries information within the brain and between the brain and other parts of the body；a nerve cell 神经元

chatty /ˈtʃætɪ/   *adj*. talking a lot in a friendly way 爱说话的；爱闲聊的；健谈的

incoming /ˈɪnˌkʌmɪŋ/   *adj*. ① recently elected or chosen 新当选的；新任的 ② arriving somewhere，or being received 正到达某地的；刚收到的

leap /liːp/   *vt*. & *vi*. to jump high or a long way 跳；跳跃；跳越

daydreaming /ˈdeɪdriːmɪŋ/	*n*. absent-minded dreaming while awake 白日梦;空想
rev /rev/	*vt*. & *vi*. to increase the number of rotations per minute (使)加快转速;(使)加速
pitch /pɪtʃ/	*n*. an area of ground that is marked out and used for playing a game such as football, cricket, or hockey 球场
swing /swɪŋ/	*vt*. & *vi*. to move backwards or forwards or from side to side while hanging from a fixed point; to make sth. do this (使)摆动;摇摆;摇荡
bat /bæt/	*n*. a piece of wood with a handle, made in various shapes and sizes, and used for hitting the ball in games such as baseball, cricket and table tennis 球棒;球拍;球板
break /breɪk/	*n*. a short period of time when you stop what you are doing and rest, eat, etc. 间歇;休息
cement /səˈment/	*vt*. ① to join two things together using cement, glue, etc. （用水泥、胶等)粘结,胶合　② to make a relationship, an agreement, etc. stronger 加强,巩固(关系等)
boost /buːst/	*vt*. & *vi*. ① to make sth. increase, or become better or more successful 使增长;使兴旺　② to increase or raise 增强,提高

Phrases and Expressions

have sth. in common	有共同点
the same is true	也是如此
when it comes to	当提到
get into the act	参加
be made up of	由……组成
move away	离开;移走
in a sense	在某种意义上;有一点儿
get ready to do sth.	准备好做……
at the same time	与此同时

Text Notes

1. quiz bowl 指"机智问答"。
2. Practice makes perfect 是谚语,意为"熟能生巧"。
3. No more,即 not any more,意为"不再如此了,情况已经有所改变"。
4. 此句中,句子主干为 Bergstrom stresses the importance of sleep,而 needed to gain knowledge 为分词作定语修饰 memories,整句意为"伯格斯特龙强调了睡眠对于形成新的记忆的重要性,而这种新的记忆是获得知识所必需的"。

Text Comprehension

Please read the following statements and mark T/F according to the text.

1. Training is a common point between musicians, athletes and quiz bowl champions.

A. T   B. F
2. Doing something repeatedly can make it much easier.
   A. T   B. F
3. Recent data shows that the brain goes on changing over the course of our lives.
   A. T   B. F
4. Neurons are nerve cells and they are talkative.
   A. T   B. F
5. The more efficient the cells in a brain area related to certain task are, the less energy they use to chat.
   A. T   B. F

Vocabulary and Structure

Please complete the following sentences with the proper forms of the words given.
·1. At the age of five he showed exceptional talent as a _____. (music)
2. All newbies are offered an individually tailored _____ and development program. (train)
3. Relax as much as possible and keep breathing _____. (steady)
4. His fan base is _____ middle-aged ladies. (most)
5. My neighbour's very _____ — she tells me all the news. (chat)

Translation

Please translate the following passage into Chinese.

The brain doesn't shut down overnight. In fact, catching some zzz's can dramatically improve learning. That's because as we sleep, our brains store memories and new information from the previous day. So a poor night's sleep can hurt our ability to remember new things.

▪▪ Further Study

(Blame and Complaint)

Communication Skills

责备和抱怨(Blame and Complaint):责备和抱怨是社交中不可避免的场景。西方人说话比较直率。对于别人的打扰,自己受到的不公平待遇会以"提醒""明确表示"等方式说出来,但是不会不留面子。一般对责备与抱怨,人们通常的反应是表示抱歉(I'm sorry)与愿意接受。

Key Sentences

◆ Expressing blame and complaint
○ He is to blame.

○ You might at least have avoided doing that.

○ I'm afraid I have a complaint to make about the service.

○ You ought to be ashamed of what you've done on me.

○ You ought to be careful enough next time.

○ What on earth is the matter here?

○ What do you mean by doing so?

○ What on earth is the matter?

○ Why didn't you tell me the truth earlier?

○ Why don't you do something about it?

◆ Response

○ I'm sorry to have said that，but...

○ It's my fault.

○ I am to blame.

Practice

1. — I really hate waiting.

    — _____ . I had something urgent just now.

  A. No more   B. Excuse me

  C. I'm sorry   D. Never again

2. — I'm not at all pleased by your negligence.

    — _____ .

  A. We felt terribly sorry   B. Fine，thank you

  C. Very well   D. Not too bad

3. — Sorry. I'll make it up to you someday.

    — _____ .

  A. My pleasure   B. Very well

  C. You are all talk and no action   D. Nice to meet you

4. — I'm tired of your complaints.

    — Just listen to me. _____ .

  A. I'm serious   B. What a pleasure

  C. I don't know   D. Thanks a lot

5. — You should get used to the new job soon.

    — _____ .

  A. I don't know   B. I'm serious

  C. Not at all   D. That's easy for you to say

Grammar

强调句(Emphatic Pattern)：这是一种修辞，是人们为了表达自己的意愿或情感而使用的一种形式。通过各种方式对句子中的某个部分进行强调，从而起到修辞的作用。

英语常用的强调结构是"It is（was）+ 被强调部分（主语、宾语或状语）+ who（that）..."。一般说来，被强调部分指人时，用 who；指事物时用 that，但 that 也可以指人。

一、陈述句的强调句型

句型为：It is / was + 被强调部分（通常是主语、宾语或状语）+ that / who（当强调主语且主语指人）+ 其他部分。例如：

It was yesterday that he met Li Ping.

他在昨天见到了李萍。

二、一般疑问句的强调句型

句型同上，只是把 is / was 提到 it 前面。例如：

Was it yesterday that he met Li Ping?

他是昨天见到李萍的吗？

三、特殊疑问句的强调句型

句型为：被强调部分（通常是疑问代词或疑问副词）+ is / was + it + that / who + 其他部分？例如：

When and where was it that you were born?

你是何时何地出生的？

四、not ... until ... 句型的强调句

句型为：It is / was not until + 被强调部分 + that + 其他部分。例如：

普通句：He didn't go to bed until / till his wife came back.

强调句：It was not until his wife came back that he went to bed.

直到他妻子回来，他才睡觉。

注意：

此句型只用 until，不用 till。但如果不是强调句型，till，until 可通用；因为句型中 It is / was not ...已经是否定句了，that 后面的从句要用肯定句，切勿再用否定句了。

五、谓语动词的强调

It is / was ... that ... 结构不能强调谓语，如果需要强调谓语时，用助动词 do / does 或 did。例如：

Do sit down.

务必请坐。

Do be careful when you cross the street.

过马路时，务必（千万）要小心啊！

注意：

此种强调只用 do / does 和 did，没有别的形式；过去时用 did，后面的谓语动词用原形。

Practice

1. It was the next morning _____ he woke up.
   A．when
   B．that
   C．as
   D．which

2. _____ that caused him to serve dinner an hour later than usual.
   A．It was we being late
   B．It was we were too late
   C．It was our being late
   D．It was because we were late

3. It was _____ she was about to go to bed _____ the telephone rang.

A. when；when   B．that；that

C．when；that   D．that；when

4. _____ was very _____ that little Jim wrote the letter.

A．It；careful   B．He；careful

C．It；carefully   D．He；careful

5. It may have been at Christmas _____ John gave Mary a handbag.

A．before   B．that

C．who   D．when

Writing

失物招领（Lost and Found）：失物招领启事正文部分要求简明扼要、句式正确，对物品的描述要清晰到位、衔接自然，以便有效地将信息传达给读者。启事的最后不要忘记署名。招领启事以Found作为标题放在启事正上方。正文通常包括以下几部分：拾到物品的时间、地点及当时的情形；描述拾到物品的特征；提供详细且准确的联系方式或联系地址。

Practice

Instructions：_You have found an electronic dictionary and want to return it to its owner. Write a notice of **Found** to clearly state_：

1. the time and place of your finding；

2. the feature of the dictionary；

3. your information for contact.

Key to Exercises

Unit One

Text A

【Text Comprehension】

1. B 2. A 3. D 4. C 5. B

【Vocabulary and structure】

1. B 2. D 3. B 4. A 5. C

【Comprehensive Exercise】

1. D 2. A 3. C 4. E 5. B

【Translation】

1. 联合国已经呼吁国际社会提供援助。

2. 他一生的时间都在同种族主义和偏见做斗争。

3. 与朋友们分离使他很伤心。

4. 他从未放弃过对读书的热爱。

5. 维修这座房子花费巨大。

Text B

【Text Comprehension】

1. B 2. B 3. B 4. A 5. A

【Vocabulary and structure】

1. misunderstanding 2. willing 3. connection 4. likely 5. acquaintance

【Translation】

　　研究显示快乐的关键在于拥有一份亲密的关系以及一张朋友网络。我们的社群关系能让我们更健康，并更具有承受压力的弹性。因此要维系持续又健康的友谊是值得努力的！

Further Study

【Communication Practice】

1. A 2. C 3. B 4. B 5. C

【Grammar Practice】

1. B 2. A 3. D 4. B 5. D

【Writing Practice】

Dear Prof. Robin，

　　I am writing on behalf of the English Department to invite you to give a lecture in our college.

We know that you are an expert on British literature. We would be very grateful if you could give a lecture on "Contemporary British Literature" to the English Department on Sunday，April 8. If this subject does not suit you，any other similar topic would be welcome as well.

We sincerely hope you can come. If it is convenient for you，would you please drop me a line to let me know whether you can come or not? We could be looking forward to the opportunity to benefit from your experience and wisdom.

Sincerely yours，

Thomas Johnson

▓ Unit Two

Text A

【Text Comprehension】

1. B   2. A   3. A   4. D   5. B

【Vocabulary and structure】

1. B   2. C   3. C   4. A   5. C

【Comprehensive Exercise】

1. B   2. E   3. A   4. C   5. D

【Translation】

1. 教育是一个民族对未来最佳的投资。

2. 对于任何数量的捐赠我们都不胜感激,并会好好地利用。

3. 请正确处理电池,不要丢进火中或置于高温中。

4. 即使我们在工作中取得了很大的成绩,也不应该自满。

5. 他们不太了解如何分享与合作。

Text B

【Text Comprehension】

1. B   2. A   3. B   4. B   5. A

【Vocabulary and structure】

1. persistence   2. shortly   3. locker   4. skinny   5. tackle

【Translation】

这个年轻人的体型只有其他男孩的一半,他绝对不可能成功。他决心每次训练都全力以赴。或许他资历老些的时候会有机会上场。他像球星一样跑,传,拦截,处理球。他的队伍开始胜利了。比赛的最后关键几秒,他拦截住对方的一次传球,并且全速奔跑,为本方赢下了最后胜利的触地得分。

Further Study

【Communication Practice】

1. A   2. C   3. B   4. B   5. A

【Grammar Practice】

1. B   2. A   3. C   4. A   5. D

【Writing Practice】

Dear Mike，

　　It gives me great pleasure to be invited to attend your graduation ceremony on June 30th in the Shane Hall in our university. I would like to accept your warm invitation but I cannot due to an earlier appointment.

　　Two weeks ago，I made an appointment with one of my former colleagues，Professor Wu Hui，who would come to China to make an academic research. He asked me for help and I have consented. We are going to leave Beijing on June 25th.

　　Therefore，I feel terribly sorry for being unable to attend the event. I wish the graduation ceremony a success.

　　Sincerely yours

　　Wang Lei

▓ Unit Three

Text A

【Text Comprehension】

1. C **2.** C **3.** A **4.** C **5.** C

【Vocabulary and structure】

1. D **2.** A **3.** B **4.** C **5.** D

【Comprehensive Exercise】

1. C **2.** B **3.** E **4.** D **5.** A

【Translation】

1. 我对那个五星级酒店中服务员的礼貌举止印象深刻。

2. 勺子就在叉子的旁边。

3. 他讲话的样子好像他是老师。

4. 我来晚了仅仅是因为车坏了。

5. 礼仪能把女人装点成淑女，能让男人变成绅士。

Text B

【Text Comprehension】

1. A **2.** B **3.** B **4.** B **5.** A

【Vocabulary and structure】

1. graduation **2.** wearing **3.** meeting **4.** Eating **5.** fatter

【Translation】

　　每个大学生都期待毕业典礼。在这重要的一天，学生最想体验的是幸福感和成就感。穿礼服和戴毕业帽是毕业典礼上的一种传统。因此，毕业帽和礼服被认为是成就的象征并受到人们的尊敬。

Further Study

【Communication Practice】

1. D **2.** A **3.** B **4.** C **5.** A

【Grammar Practice】

1. B　**2.** D　**3.** C　**4.** D　**5.** A

A visit to Liaoning Museum

It was Sunday yesterday. My class went to Liaoning Museum as planned. To our surprise, there were so many people in the museum because of the special show of Riverside Scene at Qingming Festival. The painting is such a wonder. It is 528 cm long, 24.8 cm high. It tells the life of people in Song Dynasty. The painting tells us the global view of the capital city and the richness and happiness of the people at that time. I was deeply moved by the bright color and the story told by the masterpiece.

▓ Unit Four

Text A

【Text Comprehension】

1. B　**2.** B　**3.** C　**4.** B　**5.** C

【Vocabulary and structure】

1. D　**2.** A　**3.** B　**4.** A　**5.** C

【Comprehensive Exercise】

1. D　**2.** E　**3.** A　**4.** C　**5.** B

【Translation】

1. 大家都感到有些渴。

2. 与这个审判有关的所有证据必须交给警察。

3. 我们总会收到这样的提醒:要减少脂肪的摄入量。

4. 肥胖是引发多种疾病的主要因素。

5. 他既能说英语,也能说西班牙语。

Text B

【Text Comprehension】

1. A　**2.** A　**3.** B　**4.** B　**5.** A

【Vocabulary and structure】

1. addictive　**2.** excluding　**3.** tolerance　**4.** satisfaction　**5.** effectively

【Translation】

强迫性进食,有时也被称为食物成瘾,其特点是强迫或强制进食。如果听之任之,强迫性进食会导致严重的疾病,包括高胆固醇、糖尿病、心脏病、高血压、睡眠呼吸暂停和抑郁症。此外,长期的负面影响还包括肾脏疾病、关节炎、骨骼退化和脑卒中(中风)。

Further Study

【Communication Practice】

1. B　**2.** C　**3.** C　**4.** A　**5.** C

【Grammar Practice】

1. C　**2.** B　**3.** D　**4.** B　**5.** A

【Writing】

1. E　**2.** D　**3.** A　**4.** B　**5.** C

■ Unit Five

Text A

【Text Comprehension】

1. B　**2.** A　**3.** B　**4.** D　**5.** C

【Vocabulary and structure】

1. A　**2.** B　**3.** A　**4.** D　**5.** A

【Comprehensive Exercise】

1. C　**2.** B　**3.** D　**4.** A　**5.** E

【Translation】

1. 2月份他接手了前任校长的工作。

2. 锻炼有助于防止发胖。

3. 我们必须想办法限制自己的开销。

4. 她坐下来并做了几个深呼吸让自己平静下来。

5. 自从开始新的工作后，她就一直感觉压力很大。

Text B

【Text Comprehension】

1. A　**2.** B　**3.** B　**4.** B　**5.** A

【Vocabulary and structure】

1. prioritize　**2.** performance　**3.** daily　**4.** excels
5. organized　**6.** initiative　**7.** action　**8.** specific

【Translation】

　　运动是压力管理的一种有效活动，所以任何使你更活跃的事情同时也能使你感到压力减少。健身追踪器的好处在于仅仅追踪你的健身情况就能助你增加运动量；看见当天你走的步数，或运动时间，或步行的英里数能激发你多运动一点儿。

Further Study

【Communication Practice】

1. B　**2.** A　**3.** A　**4.** D　**5.** A

【Grammar Practice】

1. D　**2.** D　**3.** D　**4.** C　**5.** C

【Writing】

Flights at Beijing International Airport

　　The table displays arrivals at Beijing International Airport. It gives flight times, numbers and gates. As can be seen from the table, most flights arrived on time, but some fights were delayed.

　　Why were some flights delayed? It might be caused by some unpredicted weather changes, passengers' misuse of facilities on the planes, improper manipulation of planes, prolonged mechanic maintenance, engine problems, etc. Some causes are controllable while others are not.

To realize arrivals on time, all people, including crew members, passengers and others related, should enhance their awareness of safety and cooperation before and during flights. Policies and laws about flight safety should be enacted strictly. More detailed policies should be enforced.

■■ Unit Six

Text A
【Text Comprehension】
1. D 2. A 3. C 4. C 5. A
【Vocabulary and structure】
1. A 2. C 3. D 4. C 5. A
【Comprehensive Exercise】
1. C 2. B 3. D 4. A 5. E
【Translation】
1. 他小时候曾被严重虐待。
2. 最后萨拉终于在机场和她的孩子们再度团聚。
3. 要想得到工作许可,你必须拥有居民身份。
4. 国内舆论已转而反对战争。
5. 这家公司需要政府提供更多的财政援助。

Text B
【Text Comprehension】
1. B 2. B 3. A 4. B 5. A
【Vocabulary and structure】
1. malnutrition 2. fertility 3. maternal 4. insufficiently 5. deficiency
【Translation】
1949 年后,卫生部负责所有卫生保健活动,制定卫生政策并监督其各个方面。除协调全国、省、地方医疗设施外,卫生部还协调工业、国有企业医院和其他满足企业内员工卫生需求的网络。1981 年,这个附加的网络提供的卫生服务量占全国总量的 25% 左右。

Further Study
【Communication Practice】
1. A 2. B 3. D 4. A 5. C
【Grammar Practice】
1. A 2. C 3. A 4. D 5. C
【Writing】

Unbalanced Development of Mobile Phone Users

The bar graph demonstrates the changes of the numbers of mobile phone users per 1,000 people in the east, west and north during the four quarters. All in all, most users were in the east and users in the west accounted for the smallest percentage. The unbalanced development of mobile phone users is shown in the graph.

The main possible reason for the unbalanced development was different economic development in the three parts that year. There is faster economic development in the east than in the west and north. People in better financial situation tend to buy more mobile phones. Thus there were more mobile phone users in the east than in the west and north.

To solve the problem of unbalanced development of mobile phone users，more importance should be attached to economic development in the west and north.

▌▌ Unit Seven

Text A

【Text Comprehension】

1. B **2.** D **3.** C **4.** D **5.** B

【Vocabulary and structure】

1. A **2.** B **3.** C **4.** D **5.** C

【Comprehensive Exercise】

1. C **2.** E **3.** A **4.** B **5.** D

【Translation】

1. 事实上，他比他父亲高了好几英尺。

2. 正要进屋时，他发现自己忘记带书了。

3. 对于敌人的进攻，他们无能为力。

4. 我上学期数学没及格。

5. 医院里全是流感病人。

Text B

【Text Comprehension】

1. A **2.** B **3.** B **4.** B **5.** B

【Vocabulary and structure】

1. unventilated **2.** politician **3.** enlist **4.** crowded **5.** drainage

【Translation】

弗洛伦斯提出了在当时颇为革命性的理论，即只要改进并维护医院设施，医院的死亡率就会大幅降低。她很快成了医院建设方面的专家，全世界的医院都根据她的设计而建。弗洛伦斯·南丁格尔成功了。南丁格尔式的医院将在全世界范围内建立。

Further Study

【Communication Practice】

1. A **2.** B **3.** D **4.** C **5.** C

【Grammar Practice】

1. D **2.** B **3.** D **4.** C **5.** A

【Writing】

The Number of Car Accidents in 2006

From the graph，we can tell that there were two peaks of car accidents in 2006. One was in Feb. with the number of 32. The other was in August and the number was 39. From August，the number of car accidents had been decreasing until it reached the lowest point of the year in

December.

From the graph，we can see，two peaks happened in the most rainy seasons，spring and summer. Driving becomes more dangerous because of the slippery road. Maybe the weather is the most important reason for the car accidents.

Please be careful when you drive in rainy days.

■: Unit Eight

Text A

【Text Comprehension】

1. D **2.** B **3.** C **4.** D **5.** A

【Vocabulary and structure】

1. C **2.** D **3.** C **4.** A **5.** D

【Comprehensive Exercise】

1. D **2.** E **3.** C **4.** A **5.** B

【Translation】

1. 对此问题的争论一直没有间断过。

2. 过去我家乡的房子多由木料制成。

3. 教授走出了大厅，助手们紧随其后。

4. 由于不知道他的地址，我无法给他写信。

5. 他乔装打扮没被认出来。

Text B

【Text Comprehension】

1. A **2.** A **3.** A **4.** B **5.** A

【Vocabulary and structure】

1. musician **2.** training **3.** steadily **4.** mostly **5.** chatty

【Translation】

夜里大脑并不会停止工作。事实上，睡眠有助于明显地提高学习质量。这是因为当我们睡觉时，大脑会存储前一天的记忆和新的信息。因此，低质量的睡眠会使我们记新事物的能力大打折扣。

Further Study

【Communication Practice】

1. C **2.** A **3.** C **4.** A **5.** D

【Grammar Practice】

1. B **2.** C **3.** C **4.** C **5.** B

【Writing】

Found

On the evening of January 15th，2015，I found an electronic dictionary in the English reading-room on the 3rd floor of the new library in the east district of our university. The electronic dictionary can be generally described as follows. It is brand new and metallic gray in color. What's more，the portable electronic dictionary is as big as a piece of cake and as thin as a regular magazine.

The owner of the electronic dictionary may contact me now. My room phone number and mobile phone number are × × × × × × × × and × × × × × × × × × × × respectively. Please make appointment in advance.